NEUROSCIENCE RESEARCH PROGRESS

AUTISM SPECTRUM DISORDERS

EARLY SIGNS, INTERVENTION OPTIONS AND FAMILY IMPACT

NEUROSCIENCE RESEARCH PROGRESS

Additional books in this series can be found on Nova's website under the Series tab.

Additional e-books in this series can be found on Nova's website under the e-book tab.

NEUROSCIENCE RESEARCH PROGRESS

AUTISM SPECTRUM DISORDERS

EARLY SIGNS, INTERVENTION OPTIONS AND FAMILY IMPACT

ARLENE VALDEZ
EDITOR

NOVA BIOMEDICAL

New York

Library of Congress Cataloging-in-Publication Data

ISBN: 978-1-63482-547-4
Library of Congress Control Number: 2015936097

Published by Nova Science Publishers, Inc. † New York

Contents

Preface

Autism spectrum disorders (ASD) is a neurodevelopmental disorder characterized by impairments in communication and social skills, and marked by restricted and repetitive behaviors. In recent years, there has been an increasing growth in the prevalence of ASD with 1 in 68 children in the USA diagnosed with the disorder. The authors examine the practices for identifying early markers for ASD and in turn diagnosing the disorder. Furthermore, the interactions between genes and environments are now regarded as the most probable explanation for autism spectrum disorders (ASDs). This book includes research on the principal role infantile zinc- and mangesium-deficiency and/or toxic metal burdens play as environmental factors in the pathogenesis of autism spectrum disorders. Other chapters include research on the Family-Centered Transition Planning (FTCP) approach for ASD and the results that have been achieved by students and families; the experiences of adults with autism spectrum disorders with a focus on their social relationships; cognitive behavior therapy (CBT) in adults with high functioning ASD and ways to enhance school-based interventions for children with high-functioning autism spectrum disorders (HFASD).

Chapter 1 – With a growth in prevalence rates of Autism Spectrum Disorder (ASD), there is an increasing need for early screening for ASD in children and infants. Given the serious impairments associated with ASD and the empirical support for early intensive intervention, it is imperative that children at risk for ASD are identified early thus impacting the onset of treatment. This chapter will explore international screening practices in relation to broadband and ASD-specific screeners. A number of early detection screening instruments designed to detect ASD in the general population have been developed. Children who have siblings with ASD are at a higher risk of being diagnosed with the disorder than children in the general population. Researchers have developed specific screening tools for siblings at risk for ASD. The chapter will provide a review of practices and screening tools in the area of early diagnosis in ASD. Specific early detection screening instruments for use within the general population and with those considered biologically at risk will be reviewed in relation to research outcomes, sensitivity, specificity and predictive value. Implications for early screening will also be discussed.

Chapter 2 – The interactions between genes and environments are now regarded as the most probable explanation for autism spectrum disorders (ASDs). In this chapter, based on the results of a cohort metallomics study in which scalp hair concentrations of 26 trace elements were examined for 1,967 autistic children (1,553 males and 414 females) aged 0-15 year-old, the authors overview the epigenetic roles of infantile mineral imbalances in the aetiology of ASDs.

Five-hundred and eighty-four (29.7%), 347 (17.6%) and 114 (5.8%) was estimated deficient in zinc, magnesium and calcium, respectively, and 2.0% or less in the other essential metals. The prevalence of mineral deficiency was higher in infants aged 0-3 year-old: zinc deficiency was detected in 43.5% in male and 52.5% in female subjects. In contrast, 339 (17.2%), 168 (8.5%) and 94 (4.8%) individuals were suffered from high burden of aluminium, cadmium and lead, and 2.8% or less from mercury and arsenic.

High toxic metal burdens also were frequently detected in the infantile subjects, and high significant correlations of toxic metal burdens to zinc deficiency were observed. These findings suggest that infantile zinc- and magnesium-deficiency and/or toxic metal burdens seem epigenetically play principal roles as environmental factors in the pathogenesis of autism spectrum disorders and that metallomics approach lead to early screening and intervention of the neurodevelopment disorders. Furthermore, it has been demonstrated that there is another critical factor "infantile time window" which is essential for neurodevelopment and probably for intervention/therapy. Thus, early assessment of mineral imbalances for autistic infants including suspects would lead to early diagnosis and evidence-based nutrition therapy for the children with neurodevelopment disorders.

Chapter 3 – Studies of transition outcomes have consistently documented disappointing employment and community living outcomes for individuals with an autism spectrum disorder (ASD). To some extent, the poor transition outcomes for individuals on the autism spectrum can be attributed to poor quality transition planning. Many planning processes are driven more by a concern for compliance with regulations than by a strong desire to ensure students leave high school prepared to achieve an expansive vision of adult life.

A key feature of high quality transition planning is the active involvement of the individual and their family in the process. Families play a major role in socializing children to the norms and values of adulthood, but the process is also to some degree collaborative, as emerging adults also socialize their parents, and parents socialize each other. Thus, goals are set and decisions made jointly by students and their parents. Transition planning is most effective when it takes advantage of and builds upon these efforts, rather than supplanting them with a professionally-driven approach in which youth and families are only marginally involved. Individuals with disabilities and their families are in the best position to know what they need.

One approach to facilitating active involvement, Family-Centered Transition Planning (FCTP), has demonstrated significantly improved outcomes over traditional transition planning. The approach uses a combination of group family training sessions and a series of individual planning meetings and assistance from a planning facilitator to work on plan implementation, including career exploration activities, work experiences, and coordinating plans with other services.

In this chapter, the authors present the FCTP approach and the results that have been achieved by students and families. They will also devote specific attention to the central role that changes in student and parent expectations play in the process, both as results of and drivers of the transition planning process, and outline a theoretical account of the key elements that lead to empowered action by students and families. Finally, the authors will report current efforts to replicate and sustain the FCTP model.

Chapter 4 – Most research in the area of autism spectrum disorders has concentrated on children and adolescents, while very few studies have been conducted on adults with autism spectrum disorders (especially those diagnosed in adulthood). The aim of this qualitative study is to explore the experiences of adults with autism spectrum disorders with a focus on their social relationships. Six of the men who participated in the study were diagnosed with autism spectrum disorders in late childhood or in their teens, while the remaining four received a diagnosis in their adulthood (up to 4 years prior to the study). The diagnoses of autism spectrum disorders were made by public local educational authorities or hospital clinics by multidisciplinary teams comprising of psychiatrists, psychologists, speech therapists, occupational therapists, and social workers. Two of them lived on their own, five were living with their parents and/or siblings and the remaining three had their own families. They were interviewed by the researchers for 1.5 hours using an in-depth semi-structured format and content analysis was used to analyse and interpret their thoughts and experiences. The themes that emerged from the analysis are: coming to terms with the diagnosis; revealing the diagnosis to their family/spouse, friends and colleagues; initiating and maintaining social relationships (challenges and facilitators); the impact of culture. This is among the first qualitative studies looking at the social experiences of adults with autism spectrum disorders. Therefore, it has certain limitations such as its constrained generalization to female adults with autism spectrum disorders or males from different cultures.

Chapter 5 – Autism spectrum disorder (ASD) is a neurodevelopmental condition marked by impairment of social interaction, social communication and restricted and repetitive stereotyped patterns of behavior, interests and activities (American Psychiatric Association, 2000). ASD symptoms cause impairment across many functioning areas and are present early in life. Individuals with ASD are vulnerable to a lot of psychiatric and neurological disorders such as depression, epilepsy, sleep disorder, anxiety disorder, and obsessive compulsive disorder. In addition, hyper- or hyposensitivity to pain, touch, movement, sound, smell, and light is often reported. Recent reports suggest that adults with ASD are unable to understand their own mental states, which could lead to difficulties in emotional regulation. As a result of these psychiatric and neurological difficulties, quality of life is often impaired in adults with ASD. Various treatments have been developed to alleviate comorbid symptoms in adults with ASD. Psychological methods designed to treat children with ASD are difficult to adapt to adult patients with ASD because they either involve parental participation or are too time-consuming. However, some studies have reported the efficacy of cognitive behavior therapy (CBT) in improving emotional regulation among adults with ASD. In addition, group settings enable social interaction and sharing experiences with others, which reduces social isolation. Group CBT is additionally beneficial in terms of increasing specific skills and minimizing dropout. This review evaluates the evidence for the group CBT in adults with high functioning ASD.

Chapter 6 – Children with high-functioning autism spectrum disorder (HFASD) present with core deficits in social communication and restricted, repetitive, and stereotyped behaviors and interests that significantly impact their functioning and warrant comprehensive interventions. The knowledge and resources required to provide comprehensive interventions presents a particular challenge to treatment providers in school settings. The current chapter describes a systematic model of training and support provided to school professionals in order to guide and assist their implementation of a manualized comprehensive school-based intervention (schoolMAX) for 6-11 year old children with HFASD across the school year. The schoolMAX program was specifically designed to target the needs of children with HFASD within a school setting via social skills groups, therapeutic activities, face-voice emotion recognition instruction, individualized daily notes, and parent training. The implementation protocol consists of a three component process that includes 1) instruction, observation, planning, and practice; 2) treatment fidelity monitoring; and 3) consultative feedback. First, didactic instruction, observation, practice, and planning are used to build school staff knowledge and proficiency and to adapt the intervention to the participating school environment. Second, treatment fidelity is monitored throughout implementation by research clinicians to ensure the intervention protocol is conducted consistently and accurately. These research clinicians monitor fidelity while also providing ongoing modeling and support. Third, regular consultative feedback on provider proficiency is delivered to school staff by the senior research team. This feedback reviews ongoing intervention fidelity, problem-solves implementation issues, and evaluates student progress. Using data from the first year of a 4-year randomized trial of schoolMAX, the current study demonstrates the success of the three component implementation model in maintaining high levels of treatment fidelity by school staff across the school year. Implications for the use of this implementation model in enhancing execution of school-based interventions are discussed.

In: Autism Spectrum Disorders
Editor: Arlene Valdez
ISBN: 978-1-63482-547-4

Chapter 1

Advances in Research on the Early Identification of Autism Spectrum Disorder

***Jennifer Holloway**,[1] *Olive Healy*,[2] *Edith Walsh*[1] *and Michelle O'Brien*[1]**
[1]National University of Ireland, Galway, Ireland
[2]Trinity College, Dublin, Ireland

Abstract

With a growth in prevalence rates of Autism Spectrum Disorder (ASD), there is an increasing need for early screening for ASD in children and infants. Given the serious impairments associated with ASD and the empirical support for early intensive intervention, it is imperative that children at risk for ASD are identified early thus impacting the onset of treatment. This chapter will explore international screening practices in relation to broadband and ASD-specific screeners. A number of early detection screening instruments designed to detect ASD in the general population have been developed. Children who have siblings with ASD are at a higher risk of being diagnosed with the disorder than children in the general population. Researchers have developed specific screening

* Correspondence address: Dr. Jennifer Holloway, School of Psychology, National University of Ireland – Galway, University Road, Galway, Ireland.

tools for siblings at risk for ASD. The chapter will provide a review of practices and screening tools in the area of early diagnosis in ASD. Specific early detection screening instruments for use within the general population and with those considered biologically at risk will be reviewed in relation to research outcomes, sensitivity, specificity and predictive value. Implications for early screening will also be discussed.

Autism spectrum disorder (ASD) is a neurodevelopmental disorder characterized by impairments in communication and social skills, and marked by restricted and repetitive behaviors. In recent years there has been an increasing growth in the prevalence of ASD, with 1 in 68 children in the USA diagnosed with the disorder (Centers for Disease Control and Prevention, 2014). Furthermore, in families where one child is diagnosed with ASD a reoccurrence rate of 18.7% has been reported in siblings (Ozonoff, Young, Carter, Messenger, Yirmiya, Zwaignebaum et al., 2010). With a growth in prevalence rates for ASD, practices for identifying early markers for ASD and in turn diagnosing the disorder are important to consider. With early detection, comes the possibility of early intervention.

Recognition of the importance of early intervention has not just focused on ASD, but rather extends to a range of childhood disorders, with researchers concluding that early detection and intervention being critical to positive prognosis (Birbeck and Drummond, 2005; Matson, Riseke and Tureck, 2011). There is a vast amount of empirical support for early intensive behavioral intervention (EIBI), with many children receiving treatment by the age of three years showing significant developmental gains (Harris and Handleman, 2000; Howlin et al., 2009; Reichow and Wolery, 2009; Rogers, 1996). Identifying children for ASD diagnosis through screening methods could potentially result in infants accessing intervention at earlier stages of life, pre-diagnosis when early symptoms are identifiable and when intervention has been proven to be most effective (MacDonald, Parry-Cruwys, Dupere, and Ahearn, 2014). Medical research has shown that the brain structure of young children is more malleable than that of adults, making learning easier in the former population. Neuroplasticity, the ability of the brain to adapt to environmental changes and thus influence behavior, is hypothesized as being maximal within the first years of life (Mundkur, 2005). As the brain has higher levels of plasticity during childhood, early access to intervention may facilitate faster acquisition of skills, which endure throughout the lifespan.

With a growing focus on early intervention, it only stands to reason that early identification of ASD becomes a focal point for research and practice. In order to receive an early diagnosis of ASD screening (i.e., assessing) for the absence and presence of specific behaviors associated with non-typical development must be carried out. Advances in ASD research on the early signs of autism has shown that ASD characteristics can be identifiable in children as young as 18 months (Bryson, Zwaignebaum, Brian, Roberts, Szatmari, Rombough et al., 2007; Garon et al., 2008; Landa et al., 2007; Ozonoff et al., 2010, Yoder et al., 2009). Deficits in communication, social deficits and higher levels of motor and object repetitive behaviors have been identified as early markers of ASD (Boyd, Odem, Humphreys and Sam, 2010) Despite the early behavioral markers identified for ASD, the current average age for a diagnosis of ASD is approximately three years or older (Mandell, Novak, and Zubritsky, 2005).

Interestingly, parents of children diagnosed with ASD often report they noticed markers for ASD well before their child was diagnosed with the disorder. Parents report early signs of ASD in their children before age three (76.2%) and 83.3% of parents have reflected that the signs were present before age two (Jonsdottir, Saemundsen, Antonsdottir, Sigurdardottie, and Olason, 2011). Furthermore, Kishore and Basu (2011) reported that 50% of parents in their study had concerns before 12 months of age. However, even when parents have noted concerns before age three, there is still a considerable delay in securing a diagnosis of ASD (Chakrabarti, 2009). This can be due to parents delaying on seeking referral for diagnosis and/or issues in relation to accessing clinicians to diagnose. Moreover, ASD symptoms once observed, tend to remain stable (Chawarska, Klin, Paul, Macari, and Volkmar, 2009), thus confirming again the importance of early intervention.

Screening Practices

Screening refers to the practice of testing individuals in the general population to identify factors that signal a potential risk for certain medical or behavioral conditions. The objective of a screening programme is to identify people that are more likely to be helped than harmed by getting a diagnosis or treatment for the condition (Al-Qabandi et al., 2011). Children who are deemed to be at risk for ASD, either by virtue of biological factors or through parental concerns, are often placed on surveillance. Surveillance refers to the practice of the specific use of diagnostic tests to confirm or not a diagnosis for individuals with a higher probability of receiving said diagnosis (Al-Qabandi et al., 2011). More specifically, children should be screened as part of routine developmental checks, with children showing markers/concerns for ASD, being put on specific surveillance programmes and/or beginning treatment.

Screening and surveillance practices differ across countries however the premise remains the same, identification of the early signs of ASD. Researchers have argued for developmental screening and surveillance to be a component of every preventive care visit (Hayes, and Healy, 2014; Johnson, Myers, and Disabilities, 2007). Practitioners should be guided by the four factors associated with development surveillance (Johnson et al., 2007). These surveillance factors include; having a sibling with ASD, parental concern (e.g.,, inconsistent hearing, unusual responsiveness), other caregiver concern and pediatrician concern. If the infant presents with two or more of these factors it is important for practitioners to assess the infant using a standardized developmental screening tool and refer the child for ASD evaluation. In addition to using the screening tools with infants at risk for ASD diagnosis, the screening tools should be used with all children at the 9, 18, and 30month developmental checks (AAP, 2006). The screening tools employed at the developmental checks capture; social- communicative impairments, visual attention impairments and sensory orientated behaviors (García-Primo et al., 2014). The individual screening tools will be discussed further in this chapter.

There have been a number of screening tools developed to test for specific early signs of ASD in young children. To date, some of these screening tools are more empirically validated than others. Screening is typically conducted at two levels. Level 1 screening (i.e., broadband developmental screening) refers to assessing children in the general population for characteristics of ASD. The tools are usually administered by general health practitioners and are considered to be somewhat brief in relation to content. The advantages of broadband screening include, the limited time necessary to administer, the limited costs associated with completing the assessments, screening for multiple developmental disorders with one tool and accessibility to the tools. However, some studies suggest the sensitivity of broadband screening warrant further investigation (Robins and Dumont-Mathieu, 2006). Level 2 screening (i.e., ASD specific screening) tools are specifically designed to assess children who are already considered "at risk" (e.g.,, referred from a health care practitioner who has concerns for the child's development or a sibling of a child with ASD who is at biological risk of the disorder). Level 2 screening tools are usually administered by specialist professionals, they are typically more time consuming as they investigate the child's development in greater depth. ASD specific screeners are usually administered to children that are considered at risk of ASD diagnosis due family history or failing the broadband screening process.

Current screening practices and early diagnosis procedures vary between the North America and Europe. There are numerous clinical recommendations set out by various organisations within North America. Specifically, The Centre for Disease Control and Prevention (CDCP; 2014) provide a list of comprehensive recommendations and guidelines. In addition, The American Academy of Pediatrics (AAP; 2006) recommends that developmental surveillance be incorporated at every well-child preventive care visit, it is stated that the early identification of developmental disorders in an integral function of all health care professionals. These organizations recommend that screening tests should be administered regularly at the 9-, 18-, and 24- or 30-month visits. The American Academy of Neurology and the Child Neurology Society (CDCP, 2014) list seven clinical practice recommendations; (1) surveillance should be performed at all well-child visits; (2) recommended developmental screening tools include the Ages and Stages Questionnaire, the BRIGANCE® Screens, the Child Development Inventories, and the Parents' Evaluations of Developmental Status; (3) use of the Denver-II (DDST-II) and the Revised Denver Pre-Screening Developmental Questionnaire (R-DPDQ) should not be used due to sensitivity and specificity issues; (4) timely follow-up investigation when the child fails to meet traditional milestones or shows signs of regression; (5) siblings of children with an ASD diagnosis require screening for ASD and language delay regardless of presence or absence of behavioral symptoms of the disorder; (6) the utility of empirically validated instruments for screening, and (7) audiologic assessment and lead screening are recommended for any child with developmental delay and/or ASD. Collaboration between the American Academy of Pediatrics (AAP), the Centre for Disease Control (CDC) and First Signs have resulted in the publication of The A.L.A.R.M. guidelines (Johnson, 2004). The guidelines were developed to establish standard practices among physicians, to simplify the screening process, and to ensure that all children receive routine and appropriate screenings and timely interventions. A.L.A.R.M is an acronym for five key practices in early detection: (1) know that autism is prevalent (A); (2) listen to parents (L); (3) act early (A); (4) refer (R), and (5) monitor (M).

In contrast, within Europe, information on the prevalence of ASD is still unwieldy across countries and this is mainly attributed to a lack of consistency in diagnostic practices and a lack of agreement on case definition (García-Primo et al., 2014). In 2005, The European Commission initiated a project titled the European Autism Information System (EAIS, 2005). Work package eight of EAIS has specifically focused on creating a harmonized early detection tool for countries within the European Union. The objective is to establish guidelines for early identification and diagnosis on the basis of a comprehensive analysis of existing tools and methodologies. Studies within this work package are on-going and to date a number of existing tools for early diagnosis have been examined (i.e., ADOS, ADI-R, CHAT, M-CHAT, CHAT23, CARS, DSMIV, ICD10). In July 2006, an ad hoc questionnaire (Q-EAIS) was designed within the framework of the EAIS Project by the ASD Study Group of the "Research Institute for Rare Diseases" in Spain. The aim of the questionnaire was to provide a better understanding of the diagnostic and screening issues faced by people diagnosed with ASD in the participating EAIS Project countries. A total of 11 questionnaires were collected (Bulgaria, Czech Republic, Denmark, England, France, Italy, Malta, Poland, Portugal, Scotland Highland Region and Spain). Every country reported that ASD cases are mainly detected at the Public Health Care System, 72% of them in the regional or national reference centre or hospital for ASD. The age at which diagnosis of autism is obtained varied, the reported averages are: 34 years old for autism (72%), 56 years old for Asperger's syndrome (36%) and 35 years old for PDD-NOS. Of all the countries surveyed, 45% state that they have a well-child surveillance protocol after 18 months and 54% report to have an established protocol at the Public Health Service for ASD early detection (Posada, García-Primo, José-Ferrari and Martín-Arribas, 2007). There is further work to be completed within this project to ensure positive outcomes for screening and survellience of ASD in Europe.

In addition, researchers within this work package have provided a comprehensive examination of the literature that pertains to the early signs of autism (Second Interim Report to the European Commission DG-SANCO, 2007). This report recommends a clear need for standardized recommendations and guidelines throughout Europe in line with practices in North America.

Level 1 Screening Tools

This chapter will examine the screening instruments specifically related to early identification of ASD in the general population (Level 1 Screening) including: The Checklist for Autism and Toddlers (CHAT; (Baron-Cohen, Allen, and Gillberg, 1992); The Modified Checklist for Autism in Toddlers (M-CHAT;Robins, Fein, Barton, and Green, 2001); The Early Screening of

Autistic Traits (ESAT; Swinkels et al., 2006), and The Pervasive Developmental Disorder Screening Test –II (PDDST-II;Siegel, 2013). The CHAT and the M-CHAT will be discussed in the most detail as they are considered to be the most widely used broadband autism screeners (Sunita and Bilszta, 2013). An overview of the ESAT and PDDST-II will also be provided.

The CHecklist for Autism and Toddlers (CHAT; Baron-Cohen et al., 1992)

The CHecklist for Autism and Toddlers (CHAT) was designed over 20 years ago to assess the core characteristics of autism in infants from 18 months. The screening tool consisting of 14 questions, divided into two sections (A and B). Section A is answered by parents and includes 9 questions. These questions investigate areas of development such as; functional play, proto-imperative pointing (i.e., pointing to ask for something), motor development), social play, social interest, pretend play, joint-attention, proto-declarative pointing (i.e., following a point) and imitation. Section B comprises of five items that are completed through observation ofthe child by the health practitioner and compared to the parental report. Administration of the CHAT takes between 10 and 15 mins (Scambler, Rogers, and Wehner, 2001). The efficacy of the CHAT for detecting ASD in both at risk children and large community samples have been evaluated in many studies (Baird et al., 2000; Baron-Cohen et al., 1992; Baron-Cohen et al., 1997; Scambler et al., 2001; Scambler, Hepburn, and Rogers, 2006). Baron-Cohen et al., (1992) conducted the preliminary study to establish if detection of ASD is possible at 18months. This study involved two groups (Group 1 and 2). Group 1 consisted of a control group of infants with an aim to collect normative data. Group 2 was considered the high risk group and the researchers predicted that they should find approximately 1.2 cases of autism within this group. At a follow up at 2.5years none of the participants of Group 1 had been diagnosed with autism. In the high risk group four infants showed signed of autism (9.75%). At follow up, the four children had a confirmed diagnosis of autism by two independent psychiatrists using DSM-III-R criteria. This initial study provides applied validity of the CHAT, it suggests that; (1) toddlers with undiagnosed autism at the age of 18 months will fail three of the key behavior listed in the CHAT as protodeclarative pointing, gaze-monotoring and pretend play, and, (2) children who lack protodeclarative pointing, or protodeclarative pointing plus pretend play, at 18 months of age will be at risk of developmental delay without autism.

Baron-Cohen et al., (1997) conducted a further larger population study to evaluate the CHAT within the general population based on the evidence from the initial study. This study involved 16,000 participants, all participants were screened using a two stage method; at 18 months and again one month later. Twelve of the 16,000 children failed three items following the initial screening and were referred for diagnosis. Ten of these participants were diagnosed with autism and continued to retain their diagnosis at 3.5 years of age. False positive during screening was 16.6% for autism however; these infants still received some other diagnosis for developmental delay.

Baron-Cohen et al., (2000) analyzed the results of the population study with a series of follow-up screenings to evaluate the sensitivity, specificity, false negatives and positive predictive value (PPV) of the CHAT as an ASD screening instrument. Sensitivity refers to the probability that someone who has the condition (autism) will test positive for it. Specificity refers to the probability that someone that does not have the condition (autism) will test negatively for it. With the administration of the CHAT in two stages a total of 74 children who went to receive an ASD diagnosis had not been recognized initially. This reduced the sensitivity of the CHAT for screening autism to the low level of 18% in the high risk group, although specificity was at 100%, there was a reported PPV of 75% and negative predictive value of 99.7% (Baron-Cohen et al., 2000). In the identification of pervasive developmental disorders the same study reported the medium and high risk groups combined. The sensitivity was low at 21.3%, specificity was high at 99.9% and a PPV of 58.8%. Baird et al., (2000) too reported on the follow up study conducted by Baron-Cohen et al., (2000), they stated in their study that the CHAT had an overall sensitivity of 38% and a specificity of 98% for identifying autism in toddlers. They too recognized that the data shows low sensitivity and low PPV of the screening tool for single administration. These studies highlight difficulties with the tool in relation to its psychometric properties.

The clinical implications of this tool as an early screening method for ASD are positive. According to the data reported, if a child meets criteria for the high risk group he or she will almost certainly go on to being diagnosed with having autism or PDD. Of the medium risk group about half or so will be diagnosed with childhood autism while most of the other will have developmental delays. The low false-positive rate means that few parents will be unnecessarily alarmed. The research shows that the detection of autism and other PDD's is possible at 18 months.

The Modified Checklist for Autism and Toddlers (M-CHAT; Robins, Fein, Barton, and Green, 2001)

The M-CHAT is an extension of the CHAT, described above. The M-CHAT like the CHAT aims to identify early signs of autism by assessing the child's attainment of developmental milestones. However, the M-CHAT differs in both its delivery and content. Robins et al., (2001) proposed to improve the sensitivity of the CHAT by; (1) increasing the age of initial screening from age from 18months to 24months, (2) lower threshold for follow up, and, (3) use a structured follow up interview with the respondents, which allows for both specificity and sensitivity. The M-CHAT includes 21 additional items and now consists of 23 yes/no questions covering areas such as sensory and motor abnormalities, attention, social, language, and communication skills derived from core symptoms of autism, as identified by professionals working with individuals with ASD. The tool can be completed by a parent and then a healthcare professional can complete the follow-up questionnaire with parents of children who present with concerning symptoms. As there is no need for a health professional to be present when the M-CHAT is being completed and is based on the child's current level of development, it is very easy for parents to fill it out in the waiting room before attending the child's developmental assessment.

Robins et al., (2001) conducted the initial study involving the use of the M-CHAT. The study aimed to determine; (a) how predictive each item is for ASD and PDD, (b) what items are failed by children with ASD, (c) how many items are failed by children with ASD, (d) if total score or a sub-score could detect ASD and, (e) the score differences between the original CHAT and the revised M-CHAT. The researchers ran a discriminative functional analysis using the original 9 items from the CHAT of the 1,233 non-autistic participants 27 were misclassified as having ASD/PDD and four children were misclassified as non-autistic when the clinical diagnosis was ASD/PDD. A cut off score of two items failed would lead to sensitivity of 87%, specificity of 98%, a PPV of 63% and NPV of 99%. Through this study Robins et al., (2001) found the M-CHAT to be reliable, the data reported supports the use of the M-CHAT as a screen for the early signs of autism.

Eaves, Wingert, and Ho (2006) administered the M-CHAT using two different scoring methods. The M–CHAT1 score was based on the six key items identified with discriminant function by Robins et al., (2001) with failure of any two items suggesting a need for follow up and probable diagnosis of ASD. The M–CHAT2 score was based on 19 out of the 23 items; any three of these suggest ASD. For the M-CHAT1 method of scoring in the sample of 82 participants, 57 screened positive for ASD, 40 of these went on to receive a clinical diagnosis of ASD. Of the 25 participants that screened negative, 12 were diagnosed with ASD. These figures lead the sensitivity of the M-CHAT1 to be set at 77% and the specificity at 43%. For the M-CHAT2 scoring method of the 82 participants 70 were screened positive, 48 were diagnosed with autism and of the 12 that screened negative 4 were diagnosed with autism. The M-CHAT2 reported in Eaves et al., (2006) increased sensitivity to 92% but lowered specificity to 27%. The findings of this study suggest that increased sensitivity lowers specificity. It may be a question of ethical judgment and social costs as to which is more desirable, increased false negatives or false positives.

Kleinman et al., (2008) conducted a large population study of the M-CHAT with an aim to investigate the PPV across a general population group, Group 1 (n = 3309) and a high risk group (Group 2) (n =484) who were either screened at intake into an early intervention service or referred from a developmental pediatrician or psychologist. The groups were screened at three different stages; baseline,telephone interview and 42-54month check-up. At baseline the PPV for Group 1 was 11%, and for Group 2 this was reported as 60%. Following the baseline assessment telephone interviews were conducted this brought the PPV of Group 1 and 2 up to 65% and 76% respectively. The 42-54 month follow-up for the M-CHAT only resulted in PPV of 38%, with the M-CHAT plus telephone interview the PPV was 59%. These figures reported support the use of a combined M-CHAT administration plus telephone interview.

A more recent study analyzing the use of the M-CHAT as a screening tool, evaluated the sensitivity, specificity, PPV and NPV of the instrument across two groups, Group 1 participants had a diagnosis of PDD (n = 54) and, Group 2, all of whom had a diagnosis of language delay or developmental delay (n = 28). The infants were assessed across two conditions; (1) failing two of the six key items and, (2) failing any three items on the tool (Snow and Lecavalier, 2008). Under the first condition the data recorded were as follows; sensitivity 70%, specificity 38%, PPV 79% and, NPV 28%. Within the second condition, sensitivity was recorded as 88%, specificity as 38%, PPV as 83% and, NPV as 50%.

In a comparison study of the CHAT and M-CHAT both screeners have been labeled as promising tools for the assessment of ASD in toddlers, upon analysing the available data Sunita and Bilszta (2013) state that the M-CHAT has slightly better senstivivity than the CHAT and is the preferred method of early screening for autism in children. Researchers such as Robins et al, also support the use of the M-CHAT over the CHAT in addressing the issue of false positives by stating that it is necessary to have false positives in order to maxamise sensitivity and such false positives are greatly reduceed following the structured telephone interview employed within the M-CHAT. It is suggested that the M-CHAT is administered at 18 and again at 24 months. It can be easily completed by parents at developmetal check-ups, as it takes less than 15 min to complete.

The Early Screening of Autistic Traits (ESAT; Swinkels et al., 2006)

The ESAT is a 14-item screening checklist for ASD completed with parent/caregivers. The questionnaire is designed for children as young as 14-months. The tool is designed to be administered by health practitioners at regular check-up visits. Failure on three or more items suggests the need for a diagnostic evaluation.

Swinkels et al., (2006) conducted a two part study with the aim of creating a robust screening instrument for identifying ASD in children 8-20months of age and to further assess the sensitivity, specificity and cut off values of the tool on an independent sample (n =34) that had previously been diagnosed with ASD. This was a retrospective study, whereby the primary caregivers were questioned about their child's behavior at 14 months. Ninety four percent of participantstested positive for ASD when the cut off value was three or more negative answers. The two children who tested negative for ASD were reported to have been typically developing up until the age of 15 months and later showed signs of regression. Although the results reported in a second study conducted by Swinkels et al., (2006) show that a four item tool can be successful in identifying signs of ASD in children as young as 14 months, it would be important to note that this may increase the number of false positives when used on the general population. It is recommended that if choosing to use the four item test that it is simply used as a pre-screening instrument with the advantage of reducing the number of children needing the full 14-item version of the ESAT test.

Dietz, Swinkels, Van Daalen, Van Engeland, and Buitelaar (2006) investigated the use of the ESAT as a two-stage protocol for screening for ASD. The research was carried out on a general population sample (*n* = 31,724) aged between 14 and 15 months. Stage 1 involved the use of the 4 item pre-assessment tool. All infants who screened positive in the initial assessment were re-evaluated in Stage 2 by using the 14-itme ESAT instrument delivered by a trained clinician. This observational assessment was conducted within the child's home. Following the observation and 14-item assessment (the cut off score of three or more negative responses was applied), these children were then considered "high risk" (*n* = 73). Of the 73 children remaining in the study, 18 were diagnosed with ASD (25%), of the remaining children within the study, 75% were considered false positives for ASD, none were typically developing, all children received some diagnosis following clinical observations and assessment. Oosterling et al., (2010) further demonstrated the utility of the tool in screening autism in children at 14-15 months old. This screening tool's utility shows promise but further investigated is necessary.

The Pervasive Developmental Disorders Screening Test-Second Edition (PDDST-II; Siegel, 2013)

The PDDST-II consists of a questionnaire designed to screen for autism in children, 12- 48 months of age. Three versions were developed for different settings, referred to as stages: Stage 1: Primary Care Screener, intended for use within the primary care setting; Stage 2: Developmental Clinic Screener is designed for use with children who are currently in receipt of developmental services; and Stage 3: Autism Clinic Severity Screener is designed to help differentiate autism from other pervasive developmental disorders. Each version is designed to take 15min, and 5min for clinicians to score. The PDDST-II manual reports the sensitivity and specificity of the test at each stage. The Stage 1- PCS uses a cut of score of 5 reporting sensitivity at 92% and specificity of 91%. The Stage 2- DCS also uses a score of 5, sensitivity is 73% and specificity is 49% at the cut off value. The Stage 3- ACSS uses a score of 8 as a cut-off point, the sensitivity is 58% and specificity is reported at 60%. It is important to note that the PDDST-II is a screening tool and not diagnostic measure even though is assesses severity of autism in Stage 3

(Montgomery, Duncan, and Francis, 2007). It is recommended that further research be carried out on the assessment in relation to reliability, as the initial studies do not show any evidence of inter-reliability measures. This particular assessment is in the early stages of evaluation and would benefit from further research to determine utility in the clinical setting (Matson, Rieske and Tureck, 2011).

Level 2 Screening, ASD Specific Screeners

Children who have siblings with ASD are at a higher risk of an ASD diagnosis than children in the general population (Bailey et al., 1995; Grice and Buxbaum, 2006). Research has found that ASD is highly inheritable and non-twin siblings have a 5-8% risk of receiving a diagnosis of ASD, with the risk increasing to 20% for the broader phenotype (American Psychiatric Association 2000; Wolff, 2004), and a 60% risk of ASD for monozygotic twins (Filipek et al., 1999). Research has shown that early signs of autism can be identified in the first 2 years of life in 'at risk' infants (Bryson et al., 2007; Garon et al., 2008; Landa et al., 2007; Ozonoff et al., 2010; Yoder et al., 2009). Early signs or markers for ASD can include deficits in communication, social skills and behavior problems. Several researchers have examined and tested screening tools for children who are at risk of diagnosis of Autism Spectrum Disorder (Bryson, Zwaigenbaum, McDermott, Rombough, and Brian 2008; Feldman, Ward, Savona, Regehr, Parker, Hudson, Penning, and Holden, 2012; Horovitz and Matson, 2013; Matson, Boisjoli, Hess, and Wilkens, 2010; Matson, Wilkens, and Fodstad, 2011; Stone, Coonrod, Turner, and Pozdol, 2004).

The next section will provide a review of specifically designed autism specific screening tools for infants deemed at risk for ASD. Such tools include, the Screening Tool for Autism in Two-Year-Olds (STAT; Stone et al., 2000), the Autism Observation Scale for Infants (AOSI; Bryson et al., 2008), the Baby and Infant Screen for Children with Autism Traits (BISCUIT; Matson et al., 2009), and the Parent Observation of Early Markers Scale (POEMS; Feldman et al., 2012).

The Screening Tool for Autism in Two-Year-Olds (STAT; Stone et al., 2000)

The Screening Tool for Autism in Two-Year-Olds (STAT; Stone et al., 1997) is an interactive screening measure that was designed for children aged from 24-35 months. The STAT was derived from three measures, The Play Assessment Scale (Fewell, 1991), the Pre-linguistic Communication Assessment (Stone, Ousley, Yoder, Hogan, and Hepburn, 1997), and the Motor Imitation Scale (Stone, Ousley, and Littleford, 1997) to differentiate children with autism from other developmental disorders. It consists of 12 interactive items for observing infant's behaviors in the areas of play, communication, and imitation skills. The STAT takes approximately 20 minutes to complete and is administered by a trained professional within a play context.

To examine the validity and to identify a scoring algorithm for the STAT that would maximize accurate identification of children diagnosed with ASD, Stone et al., (2000) compared 19 children with ASD and 54 children with non-autistic developmental disorders. Stone et al., (2000) found that the STAT had reasonable sensitivity and specificity (.83). Extending on their earlier studies Stone and colleagues used signal detection procedures to identify cut-off scores for the STAT with developmentally matched groups of 26 children with a clinical diagnosis of autism and 26 children with developmental delay and/or language impairments (Stone et al., 2004). The specificity, sensitivity and the predictive values for all were high. The inter-rater agreement and the test-retest reliability were reported at acceptable levels. To determine the utility of the STAT for children less than 24 months, Stone et al., (2008) administered the STAT to 71 high-risk children aged between 12 and 23 months old. Using an adjusted cut-off score to reflect less developed social and communication skills in the infant group, the STAT showed reasonable sensitivity (.93) and specificity (.83) for at risk infants aged 14 months and older.

Research in the area demonstrates strong psychometric properties for the STAT as a Level 2 screening measure for ASD (Stone et al., 2004). In addition to its use as a screening tool, the STAT can provide clinicians with key information on target areas for designing and developing early intervention programs (Stone et al., 2000). The STAT is a useful initial tool for screening young children for ASD and can be used not only with children at a single age but also with children covering a 12-month age range. Furthermore, research has shown that the STAT can be effective in screening children under 24 months old for ASD (Stone et al., 2008). The items on the STAT are developmentally sensitive however, may not be useful in older children as items such as specific impairments in imitation, joint attention and play measured are more likely to be present and pronounced at a younger age (Stone et al., 2000).

Children presenting with milder symptoms of ASD may be less likely to be identified by the STAT (Stone et al., 2004). The utility of the STAT has been limited to university-based clinic settings and research on the use of the STAT in home and community based settings remains to be examined (Stone et al., 2000).

The Baby and Infant Screen for Children with Autism Traits (BISCUIT; Matson et al., 2009)

The Baby and Infant Screen for Children with aUtIsm Traits (BISCUIT; Matson et al., 2009) is a well-established and researched early identification tool for ASD in children 17- 37 months (Matson et al., 2009; Matson, Wilkins, and Fodstad, 2011; Matson, Boisjoli, Hess, and Wilkins, 2010). The BISCUIT is a comprehensive tool comprised of three parts. The tool is informant based, with parents responding to items on a 3-point Likert scale in the presence of the child. Collectively, the BISCUIT assesses for early signs of ASD (Part I), symptoms of commonly occurring psychopathology in ASD (Part II) and challenging behavior (Part III).

The Baby and Infant Screen for Children with aUtIsm Traits-Part 1 (BISCUIT-Part 1; Matson et al., 2009) consists of 71 items, scored on a 3-point Likert scale. These items assess the three core impairment areas of ASD (socialization, communication, and repetitive behaviors or restricted interest). The BISCUIT-Part 2 assesses symptoms of psychopathology that are often commonly diagnosed with ASD. Part 2 is comprised of 84 items that assess for obsessive compulsive disorder, Attention Deficit Hyperactivity Disorder (ADHD), tic disorder, conduct disorder, specific phobia, and eating difficulties. The BISCUIT-Part 3 measures for co-morbid challenging behavior commonly associated with ASD. Part 3 includes 20 items assessing for the presence of self-injurious, stereotypic, aggressive and disruptive behavior

Matson et al., (2009) examined the reliability of the BISCUIT in a sample of 276 high-risk children between the ages of 13-37 months. Results demonstrated robust reliability for all three parts of the BISCUIT. Matson, Wilkins and Fodstad (2011) reported on the convergent and divergent validity of the BISCUIT-Part 1 in a sample of 1,007 children between the ages of 17-37 months. Results showed very good convergent validity between the BISCUIT-Part 1, the M-CHAT and the Personal-Social domain from the Battelle Developmental Inventory-Second Edition (BDI-2; Newborg, 2005). Sensitivity and Specificity of the BISCUIT has also been established with large samples of children (Matson et al., 2009). In order to identify the factor structure of the BISCUIT-Part 1, Matson et al., (2010) employed 1,287 children between the ages of 12-37 months. The results showed three factors that closely reflected the three core areas of impairment in ASD; communication, socialization, and stereotyped repetitive behaviors.

Matson and Tureck (2012) in a review of the current status of the BISCUIT, highlight the extent to which the BISCUIT has been researched as a screening tool for ASD in young children. The psychometric properties of the test are well established and have been examined in numerous papers (Matson et al., 2009; 2010; 2011). LoVullo and Matson (2012) examined the effects of using a few items from the BISCUIT to identify children with ASD in a sample of 2,168 high-risk children aged between 17 and 37 months with results further supporting the utility of the tool. Furthermore, the BISCUIT can be used to differentiate between autism and PDD-NOS (Matson et al., 2009). The BISCUIT is a relatively quick and easy tool to administer. The outcomes of the tool can also be used for treatment planning and evaluation of progress (Matson and Tureck, 2012).

The Autism Observation Scale for Infants (AOSI; Bryson et al., 2008)

The Autism Observation Scale for Infants (AOSI: Bryson et al., 2008) was designed to detect and monitor the early signs of autism in high-risk infants aged between 6-18 months old. It is an 18-item observational measure administered by trained professionals and takes approximately 20mins to complete. The AOSI is administered in an interactive context with the child sitting on the parent's lap across from the examiner. Target behaviors (visual tracking, orientation to name, reciprocal social smiling, differential emotional expression, imitation, visual tracking and disengagement of attention) are assessed through a series of standard play activities (e.g.,, blocks, book) with the examiner using 'systematic presses' to elicit target behaviors during the activities (Bryson et al., 2008,). To examine the inter-rater and the test-retest reliability of the AOSI, Bryson et al., (2008) examined high-risk infants, at 6, 12, and 18 months. The inter-rater agreement and test-retest reliability was acceptable, however further studies are needed.

Autism Specific Screening in Children within the First Year (0-12months)

Relatively few ASD specific screeners show promise-detecting ASD in children under 24 months. The STAT and AOSI require direct testing of the child by trained professionals and more research is warranted on these tools. Furthermore, neither instrument nor the BISCUIT have been developed to detect ASD in the first year of life.

Parent Observation of Early Markers Scale (POEMS; Feldman et al., 2012)

The Parent Observation of Early Markers Scale (POEMS: Feldman et al., 2012) was designed to detect early signs of ASD in1-24 months old infants with older siblings diagnosed with ASD. The POEMS was designed based on a review of autism assessment instruments which included the Autism Diagnostic Observation schedule-generic (ADOS-G; Lord et al., 2000), the Childhood Autism Rating Scale (CARS; Schopler et al., 1988) and the Autistic Diagnostic Interview-revised (ADI-R; Lord et al., 1994). It is a parent-report measure and includes 61 specific behaviors that include core features of ASD, such as social-communicative behaviors, restricted interests, and ritualistic and repetitive behaviors. Other items on the POEMS assess for behavioral, emotional and other problems commonly associated with young children with ASD (e.g.,, problem with eating, sleeping, transitioning, waiting, new foods, loud noises, visual tracking, attention, and movement). There are no subscales, with all items being listed by topic (e.g.,, communication, feeding).

To develop and examine the validity of the POEMS, Feldman et al., (2012) tested the tool with parents of 108 at-risk infants (74 males, 34 females). The preliminary findings show acceptable reliability and validity to warrant future research. The results showed promising predictive validity in differentiating between at-risk infants at 3-24 months of age who were later independently diagnosed with ASD at 36 months. With relatively low cut-off scores, Feldman et al., (2012) found that the POEMS had reasonable sensitivity (.74) and specificity (.73) for at risk-infants less than 24months of age. The results from Feldman et al., (2012) correspond to previous research showing that early signs of ASD may be observed as early as 9 months, if not earlier in high-risk infants (Ozonoff et al., 2010). However research is needed with a larger sample size and extended follow-up. As the sample size of children who went on to receive a diagnosis of an ASD was small (*n*=9), these results should be interpreted with caution until they are replicated in larger samples.

Routine Screening

The importance of early screening for the early identification of ASD is fundamental to the acquisition of early intervention services for young children with ASD. It is known that children make greater developmental progress in the earlier years (MacDonald et al., 2014) . The importance and necessity of broadband screening in the general population to identify ASD at the youngest possible age has been discussed. The key elements of a successful broadband screening tool have been outlined in Al-Qabandi, Gorter, and Rosenbaum (2011) as (a) being widely available, (b) simple to administer, (c) inexpensive. (d) associated with minimal discomfort to the population and, (e) producing valid and reproducible results. All Level 1 screening tools described within the chapter, meet these characteristics with exception to the limited research available on the validity of the PDDST-II. The question moreover is which is best for identifying ASD in the general population. The CHAT and M-CHAT have the most empirical support for the early identification of ASD and when compared, the M-CHAT can be the determined as the most accurate tool for early identification of ASD in children from 18 to 24 months. All children should be screened using the M-CHAT at both their 18 and 24 month developmental check-ups as routine practice (AAP, 2006). The Level 2 screening tools continue to be empirically investigated. The utility of the autism specific screening tools not only identify children at risk for ASD due to family history but can also be used as guides for the design of intervention goals. Furthermore, the tools can be used to monitor the child's developmental progress.

There is empirical support for the use of screening tools to detect early signs of ASD in children as young as 18 months and before. There is much debate as to whether early and routine screening should become common practice in infants. Al-Qabandi et al., (2011) suggest that most screening tools fail to meet a suitable standard. These suggestions link into the discussion about social costs and benefits discussed earlier in the chapter surrounding the topic of false positives and whether or not these are acceptable. False positives on screening instruments cannot be avoided in a tool with a high sensitivity power. In addition, many of the tools can be used by parents. There are a number of issues related to parent's scoring their own child's behavior and the implications for reliable assessment. Parents may incorrectly estimate their child's ability or disability and so it is important to include trained professionals in the screening and surveillance programmes. This in turn will ensure parents are offered appropriate supports and information in relation to diagnosis and treatment options. It is also important to note with all screening tools that parents and physicians should be aware of delays in communication, socialization and play behaviors that are common in childhood, rather than solely the presentation of typical autistic behaviors (Robins et al., 2001; Sunita and Bilszta, 2013).

In general the early screening tools for children are risk of ASD can only be seen as, an advancement in detection and intervention for children and their families. Although some of the screening tools require further empirical investigation, it is evident that screening and surveillance provides options to parents and healthcare workers who have identified a child as presenting with atypical developmental behavior patterns. Given the role of early intervention in the remediation of difficulties presented by children with ASD, early identification is of clinical and empirical importance.

References

Al-Qabandi, M., Gorter, J. W., and Rosenbaum, P. (2011). Early Autism Detection: Are We Ready for Routine Screening? *Pediatrics*. doi: 10.1542/peds.2010-1881

American Association of Paediatrics (2006). Identifying Infants and Young Children with Developmental Disorders in the Medical Home: An

Algorithm for Developmental Surveillance and Screening. *Pediatrics, 118*(1), 405-420. doi: 10.1542/peds.2006-1231

American Psychiatric Association (2000). Diagnostic and statistics manual of mental disorders (4th ed., text revision DSM-IV-TR). Washington, DC: Author.

Bailey, A., Le Couteur, A., Gottesman, I., et al.,. (1995). Autism as a strongly genetic disorder: evidence from a British twin study. *Psychology Medicine*, 28, 351-368.

Baird, G., Charman, T., Baron-Cohen, S., Cox, A., Swettenham, J., Wheelwright, S., and Drew, A. (2000). A Screening Instrument for Autism at 18 Months of Age: A 6-Year Follow-up Study. *Journal of the American Academy of Child and Adolescent Psychiatry, 39*(6), 694-702. doi: http://dx.doi.org/10.1097/00004583-200006000-00007

Baron-Cohen, S., Allen, J., and Gillberg, C. (1992). Can autism be detected at 18 months? The needle, the haystack, and the CHAT. [Comparative Study Research Support, Non-U S Gov't]. *Br J Psychiatry, 161*, 839-843.

Baron-Cohen, S., Cox, A., Baird, G., Swettenham, J., Nightingale, N., Morgan, K., . . . Charman, T. (1997). Psychological markers in the detection of autism in infancy in a large population. *Early Human Development, 47*(1), 98-99. doi: http://dx.doi.org/10.1016/S0378-3782(97)81293-5

Baron-Cohen, S., Wheelwright, S., Cox, A., Baird, G., Charman, T., Swettenham, J., . . . Doehring, P. (2000). Early identification of autism by the CHecklist for Autism in Toddlers (CHAT). [Research Support, Non-U S Gov't Review]. *J R Soc Med, 93*(10), 521-525.

Birbeck, D., & Drummond, M. (2005). Interviewing and listening to to the voices of, very young children on body image and perceptions of self. *Early Child Development and Care,* 176, 579-596

Boyd, B.A., Odom, S.L., Humphreys, B.P., & Sam, A.M. (2010). Infants and toddlers with Autism Spectrum Disorder: Early identification and early intervention. *Journal of Early Intervention, 32,* 73-96.

Bryson, S. E., Zwaigenbaum, L., Brian, J., Roberts, W., Szatmari, P., Rombough, V., et al.,. (2007). A prospective case series of high-risk infants who developed autism.*Journal of Autism and Developmental Disorders, 37,* 2-24.

Bryson, S. E., Zwaigenbaum, L., McDermott, C., Rombough, V., and Brian, J. (2008). The Autism observation scale for infants: Scaledevelopment and reliability data. *Journal of Autism and Developmental Disorders, 38*, 731–738.

Centre for Disease Control and Prevention (2014). Recommendations and Guidelines. Retrieved from http://www.cdc.gov/ncbddd/actearly/hcp/hcp-guidelines.html

Chawarska, K., Klin, A., Paul, R., Macari, S., & Volkmar, F. (2009). A prospective study of toddlers with ASD: Short-termdiagnostic and cognitive outcomes. *Journal of Child Psychology and Psychiatry, 50,* 1235–1245.

Chakrabarti, S. (2009). Early identification of autism. *Indian Pediatrics, 46,* 412–414.

Dietz, C., Swinkels, S., van Daalen, E., van Engeland, H., and Buitelaar, J. (2006). Screening for Autistic Spectrum Disorder in Children Aged 14–15 Months. II: Population Screening with the Early Screening of Autistic Traits Questionnaire (ESAT). Design and General Findings. *Journal of Autism and Developmental Disorders, 36*(6), 713-722. doi: 10.1007/s10803-006-0114-1

Eaves, L. C., Wingert, H., and Ho, H. H. (2006). Screening for autism: agreement with diagnosis. [Validation Studies]. *Autism, 10*(3), 229-242.

European Autism Information System (2005). Health Information. Retrieved from http://ec.europa.eu/health/archive/ph_projects/2005/action1/action1_2005_13_en.htm#3

Feldman, M. A., Ward, R. A., Savona, D., Regehr, K., Parker, K., Hudson, M., Penning, H., and Holden, J. J. A. (2012).Development and Initial Validation of a Parent Report Measure of the Behavioral Development of Infants at Risk for Autism Spectrum Disorders.*Journal of Autism and Developmental Disorders, 42,* 13-22.

Fewell, R. R. (1991). *Play Assessment Scale (5th Revision).* Unpublished manuscript, University of Miami School of Medicine.

Filipek, P. A., Accardo, P. J., Baranek, G. T., Cook, E. H., Dawson,G., Gordon, B., et al.,. (1999). The screening and diagnosis ofautistic spectrum disorders.*Journal of Autism and Developmental Disorders, 29,* 439-484.

García-Primo, P., Hellendoorn, A., Charman, T., Roeyers, H., Dereu, M., Roge, B., . . . Canal-Bedia, R. (2014). Screening for autism spectrum disorders: state of the art in Europe. *European Child & Adolescent Psychiatry, 23*(11), 1005-1021. doi: 10.1007/s00787-014-0555-6

Garon, N., Bryson, S. E., Zwaigenbaum, L., Smith, I. M., Brian, J., Roberts, W., et al.,. (2008).Temperament and its relationship toautistic symptoms in a high-risk infant sib cohort.*Journal of Abnormal Child Psychology, 37*, 59–78.

Grice, D. E., and Buxbaum, J. D., (2006). The genetics of autism spectrum disorders.*Neuromolrcular Medicine*, 8, 451-460.

Harris, S. L., and Handleman, J. S. (2000). Age and IQ at intake as predictors of placement for young children with autism: a four- to six-year follow-up. *Journal of Autism Dev Disord, 30*(2), 137-142.

Hayes, P., and Healy, O. (2014). Autism: early diagnosis key to better outcomes.Pediatrician Guide

Horovitz, M. & Matson, J. L. (2013). The Baby and Infant Screen for Children with aUtIsm Traits-Part 3: The development of age-based scoring procedures. *Research in Autism Spectrum Disorders, 9*(11), 1291-1299

Howling, P., Magiati, I., Charman, T., & MacLean, W.E. (2009). Systematic review of earli intensive behavioral interventions for children with autism. *American Journal on Intellectual and Developmental Disabilities,* 114, 23-41.

Jonsdottir, S. L., Saemundsen, E., Antonsdo ttir, I. S., Sigurdardottir, S., &O´ lason, D. (2011). Children diagnosed with autism spectrum disorder before or after the age of 6 years. Research in Autism Spectrum Disorders, 5, 175–184.

Johnson, C.P. (2004). New tool helps primary care physiscians diagnose autism early. *AAP News, 24*(2), 74.

Johnson, C. P., Myers, S. M., & Disabilities, a. t. C. o. C. W. (2007). Identification and Evaluation of Children With Autism Spectrum Disorders. *Pediatrics, 120*(5), 1183-1215. doi: 10.1542/peds.2007-2361

Kishore, M. T., & Basu, A. (2011). Early concerns of mothers of children later diagnosed with autism: Implications for early identification. *Research in Autism Spectrum Disorders, 5,* 157–163.

Kleinman, J. M., Robins, D. L., Ventola, P. E., Pandey, J., Boorstein, H. C., Esser, E. L., . . . Fein, D. (2008). The Modified Checklist for Autism in Toddlers: a follow-up study investigating the early detection of autism spectrum disorders. *Journal of Autism and Developmental Disorders, 38*(5), 827-839.

Landa, R. J., Holman, K. C., and Garrett-Mayer, E. (2007).Social and communication development in toddlers with early and later diagnosis of autism spectrum disorders. *Archives of General* Psychiatry, 64, 853–864.

Lord, C., Risi, S., Lambrecht, L., Cook, E. H., Jr., Leventhal, B. L., DiLavore, P. C., et al., (2000). The Autism diagnostic observation schedule-generic: A standard measure of social and communication deficits associated with the spectrum of autism. *Journal of Autism and Developmental Disorders, 30*(3), 205-223.

Lord, C., Rutter, M., & Le Couteur, A. (1994). Autism Diagnostic interview-revised: a revised version of a diagnostic interview for caregivers of indivduals with possible pervasive developmental disorders. *Journal of Autism and Developmental Disorders, 24,* 659-685.

LoVullo, S. V., & Matson, J. L. (2012). Development of a critical item algorithm for the Baby and Infant Screen for Children with aUtism Triats. *Research in Autism Spectrum Disorders, 6,* 378-384

MacDonald, R., Parry-Cruwys, D., Dupere, S., & Ahearn, W. (2014). Assessing progress and outcome of early intensive behavioral intervention for toddlers with autism. *Research in Developmental Disabilities, 35*(12), 3632-3644. doi: http://dx.doi.org/10.1016/j.ridd.2014.08.036

Mandell, D. S., Novak, M. M., & Zubritsky, C. D. (2005). Factors associated with age of diagnosis amoung children with autism spectrum disorders. *Pediatrics, 116*(6), 1480-1486.

Matson, J. L., Rieske, R. D., & Tureck, K. (2011). Additional considerations for the early detection and diagnosis of autism: Review of available instruments. *Research in Autism Spectrum Disorders, 5,* 1219-1326.

Matson, J. L., and Tureck, K. (2012). Early diagnosis of autism: current status of the Baby and Infant Screen for Children with aUtIsm traits (BISCUIT-Parts 1,2, and 3). *Research in Autism Spectrum Disorders, 6,* 1135-1141.

Matson, J. L., Wilkins, J., Sevin, J. A., Knight, C., Boisjoli, J. A., and Sharp, B. (2009). Reliability and item content of the Baby and Infant Screen for Children with aUtIsm Traits (BISCUIT): parts 1–3. *Research in Autism Spectrum Disorders, 3,* 336–344.

Matson, J. L., Boisjoli, J., Hess, J. A., and Wilkins, J. (2010). Factor structure and diagnostic fidelity of the Baby and Infant Screen for Children with aUtIsm Traits-Part 1 (BISCUIT-Part 1).*Developmental Neurorehabilitation, 13,* 72-79.

Matson, J. L., Wilkins, J., and Fodstad, J. C. (2011). The validity of the Baby and Infant Screen for Children with aUtIsm Traits: part 1 (BISCUIT: Part1). *Journal of Autism and Developmental Disorders, 41,* 1139-1146.

Matson, J. L., Rieske, R. D., & Tureck, K. (2011). Additional considerations for early detection and diagnosis of autism: Review of available instruments. *Research in Autism Spectrum Disorders,* 5, 1319-1326

Montgomery, J. M., Duncan, C. R., and Francis, G. C. (2007). Test Review: Siegel, B. (2004). Pervasive Developmental Disorder Screening Test—II

(PDDST-II). San Antonio, TX: Harcourt. *Journal of Psychoeducational Assessment, 25*(3), 299-306. doi: 10.1177/0734282906298469

Mundkur, N. (2005). Neuroplasticity in children. *Indian Journal of Pediatrics, 72*(10), 855-857.

Newborg, J. (2005). *Battele developmental inventory-second edition.* Itasca, IL: Riverside.

Osterling, I. J., Wensing, M., Swinkels, S.H, Van Der Gaag, R.J., Visser, J. C., Woudenberg, T., et al., (2010). Advancing early detection of autism spectrum disorder by applying an integrated two-stage screening approach. *Journal of Child Psychology and Psychiatry and Allied Disciplines, 51*, 250-258.

Ozonoff, S., Iosif, A.-M., Baguio, F., Cook, I. C., Hill, M. M.,Hutman, T., et al.,. (2010). A prospective study of the emergenceof early behavioral signs of autism.*Journal of the American Academy of Child and Adolescent Psychiatry, 49*, 258–268.

Posada, M., García-Primo, P., José-Ferrari, M., & Martín-Arribas, M.C. (2007) European Autism Information System (EAIS) Report on the 'Autism Spectrum Disorders Prevalence Data and Accessibility to Services' Questionnaire (QEAIS). *Research Institute for Rare Diseases*, Instituto de Salud Carlos III: Madrid

Reichow, B., & Wolery, M. (2009). Comprehensive synthesis of early intensive behavioral interventions for young children with autism based on the UCLA young autism project model. *Journal of Autism and Developmental Disorders, 39,* 23-41

Robins, D. L., and Dumont-Mathieu, T. M. (2006). Early Screening for Autism Spectrum Disorders: Update on the Modified Checklist for Autism in Toddlers and Other Measures. *Journal of Developmental and Behavioral Pediatrics, 27*(Suppl2), S111-S119.

Robins, D. L., Fein, D., Barton, M. L., and Green, J. A. (2001). The Modified Checklist for Autism in Toddlers: an initial study investigating the early detection of autism and pervasive developmental disorders. *Journal of Autism and Developmental Disorders, 31*(2), 131-144.

Rogers, S. (1996). Brief report: Early intervention in autism. *Journal of Autism and Developmental Disorders, 26*(2), 243-246. doi: 10.1007/bf02172020

Scambler, D., Rogers, S. J., and Wehner, E. A. (2001). Can the Checklist for Autism in Toddlers Differentiate Young Children With Autism From Those With Developmental Delays? *Journal of the American Academy of Child and Adolescent Psychiatry, 40*(12), 1457-1463. doi: http://dx.doi.org/10.1097/00004583-200112000-00017

Scambler, D. J., Hepburn, S. L., and Rogers, S. J. (2006). A two-year follow-up on risk status identified by the checklist for autism in toddlers. [Research Support, N I H , Extramural]. *J Dev Behav Pediatr, 27*(2 Suppl), S104-110.

Schopler, E., Reichler, R. J., and Renner, B. R. (1988). *The childhood autism rating scale.* Los Angeles, CA: Western Psychological Services.

Second Interim Report to the European Commission DG-SANCO (2007). Activity Report. Retrieved fromhttp://ec.europa.eu/health/archive/ph_projects/2005/action1/action1_2005_13_en.htm#3

Siegel, B. (2004). *PDDST-II: Early Childhood Screener for Autistic Spectrum Disorders*: Harcourt Assessment.

Siegel, B. (2013). Pervasive Developmental Disorders Screening Test (PDDST). In F. Volkmar (Ed.), *Encyclopedia of Autism Spectrum Disorders* (pp. 2211-2215): Springer New York.

Snow, A. V., and Lecavalier, L. (2008). Sensitivity and specificity of the Modified Checklist for Autism in Toddlers and the Social Communication Questionnaire in preschoolers suspected of having pervasive developmental disorders. [Comparative Study Evaluation Studies]. *Autism, 12*(6), 627-644.

Stone, W. L., Coonrod, E. E., andOusley, O. Y. (2000). Brief report: screening toolfor autism in two-year-olds (STAT): development andpreliminary data. *Journal of Autism Developmental Disorders, 30*, 607–612.

Stone, W. L., Coonrod, E. E., Turner, L. M.,and Pozdol, S. L. (2004).Psychometricproperties of the STAT for early autism screening.*Journal of Autism Developmental Disorders, 34*, 691–701.

Stone, W. L., McMahon, C. R., and Henderson, L. M. (2008). Use ofthe screening tool for autism in two-year-olds (STAT) forchildren under 24 months: An exploratory study. *Autism, 12,*557–573.

Stone, W. L. and Ousley, O. Y. (1997). *STAT Manual: Screening Tool for Autism in Two-Year-Olds.* Unpublished manuscripts, Vanderbilt University.

Stone, W. L., Ousley, O. Y. and Littleford, C. (1997). Motor imitation in young children with autism: What's the object? *Journal of Abnormal Child Psychology, 25,* 475-485.

Stone, W. L., Ousley, O. Y., Yoder, P. J., Hogan, K. L., and Hepburn, S. L. (1997). Nonverbal communication in 2 and 3 year- old children with autism. *Journal of Autism and Development Disorders, 27,* 677-696.

Sunita, and Bilszta, J. L. C. (2013). Early identification of autism: A comparison of the Checklist for Autism in Toddlers and the Modified

Checklist for Autism in Toddlers. [Article]. *Journal of Paediatrics and Child Health, 49*(6), 438-444. doi: 10.1111/j.1440-1754.2012.02558.x

Swinkels, S. H. N., Dietz, C., van Daalen, E., Kerkhof, I. H. G., van Engeland, H., and Buitelaar, J. K. (2006). Screening for Autistic Spectrum in children aged 14 to 15 months. I: the development of the Early Screening of Autistic Traits Questionnaire (ESAT). *Journal of Autism and Developmental Disorders, 36*(6), 723-732.

Wolff, S. (2004). The history of autism.*European Child and Adolescent Psychiatry, 13,* 201–208.

Yoder, P., Stone, W. L., Walden, T., and Malesa, E. (2009). Predictingsocial impairment and ASD diagnosis in younger siblings ofchildren with autism spectrum disorder. *Journal of Autism and Developmental Disorders, 39,* 1381–1391.

In: Autism Spectrum Disorders
Editor: Arlene Valdez
ISBN: 978-1-63482-547-4

Chapter 2

Early Assessment and Intervention of Mineral Imbalances for Autistic Children

Hiroshi Yasuda,* Ph.D.
La Belle Vie Research Laboratory, Chuo-ku, Tokyo, Japan

Abstract

The interactions between genes and environments are now regarded as the most probable explanation for autism spectrum disorders (ASDs). In this chapter, based on the results of a cohort metallomics study in which scalp hair concentrations of 26 trace elements were examined for 1,967 autistic children (1,553 males and 414 females) aged 0-15 year-old, we overview the epigenetic roles of infantile mineral imbalances in the aetiology of ASDs.

Five-hundred and eighty-four (29.7%), 347 (17.6%) and 114 (5.8%) was estimated deficient in zinc, magnesium and calcium, respectively, and 2.0% or less in the other essential metals. The prevalence of mineral deficiency was higher in infants aged 0-3 year-old: zinc deficiency was detected in 43.5% in male and 52.5% in female subjects. In contrast, 339 (17.2%), 168 (8.5%) and 94 (4.8%) individuals were suffered from high burden of aluminium, cadmium and lead, and 2.8% or less from mercury and arsenic.

* Author to whom correspondence should be addressed: E-mail: yasuda@lbv.co.jp.

High toxic metal burdens also were frequently detected in the infantile subjects, and high significant correlations of toxic metal burdens to zinc deficiency were observed. These findings suggest that infantile zinc- and magnesium-deficiency and/or toxic metal burdens seem epigenetically play principal roles as environmental factors in the pathogenesis of autism spectrum disorders and that metallomics approach lead to early screening and intervention of the neurodevelopment disorders. Furthermore, it has been demonstrated that there is another critical factor "infantile time window" which is essential for neurodevelopment and probably for intervention/therapy. Thus, early assessment of mineral imbalances for autistic infants including suspects would lead to early diagnosis and evidence-based nutrition therapy for the children with neurodevelopment disorders.

Keywords: Autism spectrum disorders; aetiology of neurodevelopment disorders; infantile zinc deficiency; toxic metal burdens; epigenetic alterations; mineral imbalance profiles; infantile time window; early assessment and intervention

1. Introduction

Clarification of the pathogenesis and effective treatment of autism spectrum disorders is one of the challenges today. Autism spectrum disorders are a group of neural development disorders characterized by impairments in social interaction and communication, and by the presence of restricted and repetitive behaviours [1,2]. Autism spectrum disorders continue to increase in prevalence up to 1 in 80 children [1-3] and are known to be highly heritable (~90%), and some related genes have been reported [4-7]. However, the underlying genetic determinants are still not clarified [1,8], and the interaction of heritable factors with uncertified lifestyle and environmental factors seem play a significant role in the pathogenesis. For example, organic mercury has been claimed one of environmental candidates causing autistic disorders [9], but its relationship remains to be not established. Recently, epigenetic alteration of gene expression by environmental factors is considered one of key events in the pathogenesis of genetic diseases [10], and some toxic elements such as cadmium and arsenic have been reported to be candidate factors that induce epigenetic alterations [11-15] and neurodevelopmental disorders [16].

For the last seven years, we have examined on the association of mineral imbalances with autistic disorders and reported that some of the autistic children have suffered from high accumulation of toxic metals such as cadmium, lead or aluminium [17-19], and in 2011 demonstrated the association with infantile zinc deficiency [20-22].

This chapter, based on the cohort metallomics study examined for 1,967 children with autistic disorders, demonstrates that many of the subjects, especially in the infants aged 0-3 year-old, are suffering from zinc- and magnesium-deficiency and/or high burdens of several toxic metals such as aluminium, cadmium, lead and so on. These findings indicate the presence of a critical term "infantile time window" in neurodevelopment and probably for therapy, suggesting that early assessment of mineral imbalances for infants is essential for early diagnosis and intervention/treatment of neurodevelopment disorders such as autism spectrum disorders and ADHD.

2. Assessment of Mineral Imbalances by Metallomics Analysis

Great advances in high-sensitive and reliable trace element analysis method using inductively coupled plasma mass spectrometry (ICP-MS) have enabled it to be applied for forensic medical researches and estimating chronic toxic metal burden and mineral deficiency in human body [23,24]. Thus, clinical applications of the reliable hair mineral analysis method with ICP-MS have been tried for investigating the association of some diseases/symptoms with the kinetics of trace elements including toxic metals and essential minerals [17,25-30], and a new omics science of "Metallomics" has been applied for investigating the pathogenesis of some genetic diseases.

We have examined the concentrations of 26 trace elements in scalp hair samples of 1,967 children with autistic disorders and discovered that many of these children are suffered from mineral imbalances [20-22]. Especially young children between 0 and 3 years-old suffered from zinc- and magnesium-deficiency and/or displayed high accumulation of toxic metals including aluminum, cadmium and lead.

The following sections exhibit that zinc- and magnesium-deficiency and toxic metal burdens are important environmental factors in the development of autistic disorders.

3. Mineral Imbalances in Autistic Children

3.1. Infantile Zinc Deficiency

Zinc is well-accepted an essential trace element that functions as the active site in more than 300 kinds of enzymes and plays important roles in nucleic acid/protein synthesis, cell replication, tissue growth and repair, especially in pregnant women and infants [31,32].

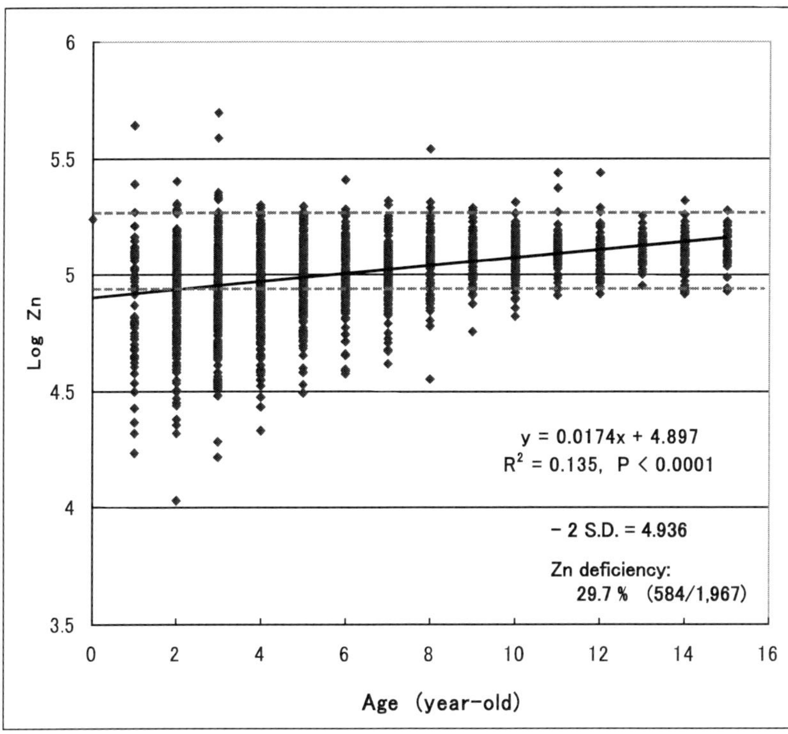

Figure 1. Age related zinc concentration in autistic children. The association of hair logarithmic zinc concentration with age in autistic children (N = 1,967) is shown [20]. Each point represents the corresponding age and logarithmic zinc concentration (ng/g hair: ppb) of the individual child. The dotted horizontal lines represent the ±2 S.D. levels of the reference range (86.3 – 193 ppm) of hair zinc concentrations. A significant relation of the zinc concentration with age ($r = 0.367$, $p < 0.0001$) in the autistic children is shown.

In brain tissue, zinc is co-stored with glutamate in pre-synaptic vesicles in the excitatory neuron terminal of hippocampus and released from the vesicles, and controls the activity of excitatory glutamate receptors on post-synaptic excitable membrane [33,34]. Thus, zinc deficiency seems associate with neurodegeneration conditions, and the initial evidence of the autism etiology linked to zinc deficiency was demonstrated in 2011 [20].

The histogram of hair logarithmic zinc concentrations for 1,967 children with autistic spectrum disorders was non-symmetric with tailing in lower range, and 584 in 1,967 subjects (29.7%) were found to have lower zinc concentration than –2 S.D. (standard deviation) level of the reference range (86.3–193 ppm; geometric mean = 129 ppm), estimated as zinc deficiency. The incidence rates of zinc deficiency in the age groups of 0-3, 4-9 and 10-15 year-old were estimated 43.5, 28.1 and 3.3% in male and 52.5, 28.7 and 3.5% in female subjects, respectively, and a significant correlation of zinc concentration with age ($r = 0.367$, $p < 0.0001$) was observed (Figure 1), suggesting that infants are more liable and susceptible to zinc deficiency than elder children and that there is a critical "infantile time window" in neurodevelopment and for intervention of autism. The minimum zinc concentration of 10.7 ppm was detected in a 2-year-old boy, corresponding to about 1/12 of the mean reference level. The zinc concentration of only one 0-year old female subject was in the normal range and seem be a suspect, because she was suffered from high burdens of aluminium (52.5 ppm), lead (9.1 ppm), iron (12.8 ppm) and copper (134 ppm). There was little marked gender difference in hair zinc concentration and incidence rate of zinc deficiency.

3.2. Infantile Magnesium/Calcium Deficiency

Next to zinc deficiency, magnesium and calcium deficiency was detected in 347 (17.6%) and 114 (5.8%) individuals in the autistic children, and for the other essential metals such as iron, chromium, manganese, copper and cobalt, their incidence rates of deficiency were 2.0% or less. The incidence rates of magnesium deficiency in the age groups of 0-3, 4-9 and 10-15 year-old were 27.0, 17.1 and 4.2% in male and 22.9, 12.7 and 4.3% in female subjects, and a significant correlation of magnesium concentration with age ($r = 0.362$, $p < 0.0001$) was observed, suggesting that infants are also liable to magnesium deficiency than elder children. The minimal magnesium concentration of 3.88 ppm was detected in a 2-year-old girl, corresponding to almost 1/10 of the mean reference level (39.5 ppm). Considerable calcium deficiency rate was observed only in lower age groups less than 10 year-old.

These finding suggest that autistic children are susceptible to deficiency in magnesium and calcium next to zinc, but not in the other essential metals such as iron and copper [21,22], and that probably infants generally have a characteristic liable to zinc- and magnesium-deficiency, because larger amounts of these trace elements (per kg body weight) are needed for the development and growth.

3.3. Toxic Metal Burdens

In contrast to essential metals, high toxic metal burdens of aluminium, cadmium and lead of over their +2 S.D. levels were observed in 339 (17.2%), 168 (8.5%) and 94 (4.8%) individuals, and the incidence rates of their burden were higher than that of mercury and arsenic (2.8 and 2.6%, respectively). High toxic metal burdens were more frequently observed in the infants aged 0-3 year-old: that is, the incidence rate was 20.6, 12.1, 7.5, 3.2 and 2.3% for aluminium, cadmium, lead, arsenic and mercury. The detected maximal concentration of aluminium, cadmium, lead, mercury and arsenic was 79.4 ppm, 5.47 ppm, 24.9 ppm, 36.3 ppm and 1.7 ppm, corresponding to 21-, 782-, 57-, 9.3- and 33-fold of each mean reference level.

Interestingly, a high significant inverse relationship between zinc and lead concentrations ($r = -0.339$, $p < 0.0001$) (Figure 2), and also aluminium ($r = -0.247$) and cadmium ($r = -0.198$) concentrations, has been observed, suggesting that these toxic metal burdens associate with zinc deficiency. There was little correlation between zinc and mercury ($r = 0.069$) or arsenic ($r = -0.143$).

In addition, a significant inverse relationship has been found between magnesium/calcium and arsenic concentration in autistic children ($r = -0.273/-0.300$). Thus, deficiency in magnesium/calcium seems enhance the accumulation and toxic effect of arsenic in autistic children.

Recently, some of toxic elements such as cadmium and arsenic have been reported to be candidate factors that induce epigenetic alterations of gene expression [11-15], and the epigenetic alteration by environmental factors is considered one of key events in the pathogenesis of genetic diseases [10] and neurodevelopmental disorders [16]. Thus, toxic metal burdens seem epigenetically play a principal role in the pathogenesis of autism and neurodevelopment disorders [16,21,22].

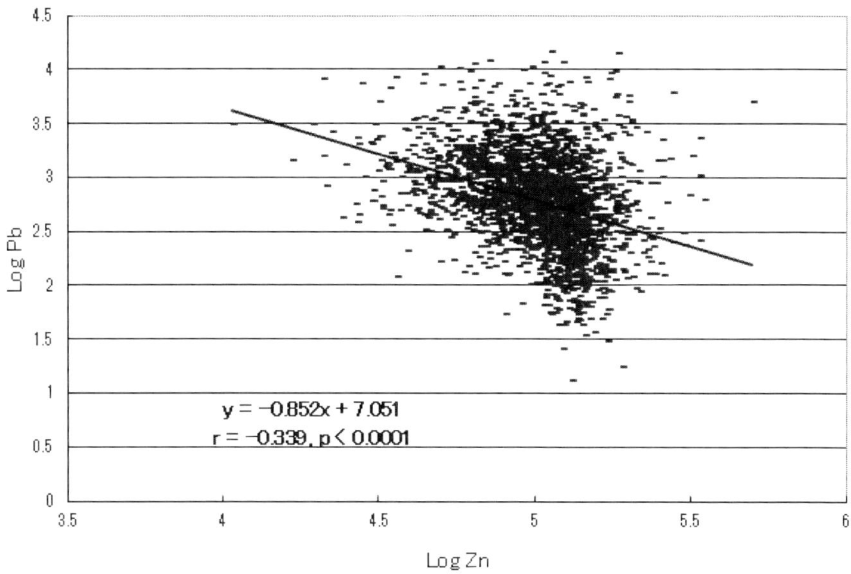

Figure 2. Inverse relation between zinc and lead concentration in autistic children. The inverse relationship between hair logarithmic zinc and lead concentration in autistic children (N = 1,967) is shown [22]. Each point represents the corresponding logarithmic zinc and lead concentration of the individual child. A high significant inverse relationship between zinc and lead concentrations ($r = -0.339$, $p < 0.0001$) in the autistic children is shown.

3.4. Mineral Imbalance Profiles in Autistic Children

Various types of mineral imbalance profiles characteristic in autistic children have been demonstrated by metallomics analysis. Figure 3 shows a typical autistic profile in a 1-year-old boy suffering from severe zinc- and magnesium-deficiency and simultaneous high burdens of cadmium and lead. The other autistic imbalance profiles with high burdens of aluminium, mercury or arsenic are shown in Figure 4-6. Figure 7 shows a unique imbalance profile with high sodium and potassium concentrations, a characteristic profile detectable in hair specimens, but not in blood plasma/serum samples. This profile appears to associate with irritable, stressful conditions of the autistic subjects with excited adrenal cortex stimulation. Thus, a variety of spectrum disorders of autism may be explained by various profile types of the mineral imbalances in bodies. It remains to be clarified which profile of these mineral imbalances does correspond to which type of autism spectrum disorders.

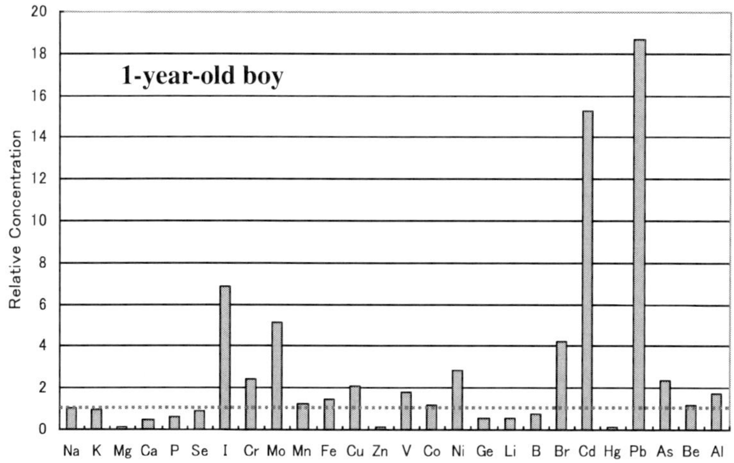

Figure 3. Mineral imbalance profile of autistic child with low zinc/magnesium and high cadmium/lead levels. A typical metallomics profile of a 1-year-old boy with autism is shown, exhibiting severe zinc- and magnesium-deficiency and simultaneous high burdens with cadmium (107 ppb) and lead (8.11 ppm) [21]. Each bar represents the relative concentration of the respective trace element in his scalp hair specimen. The dotted horizontal line at 1.0 represents the reference control level of each trace element.

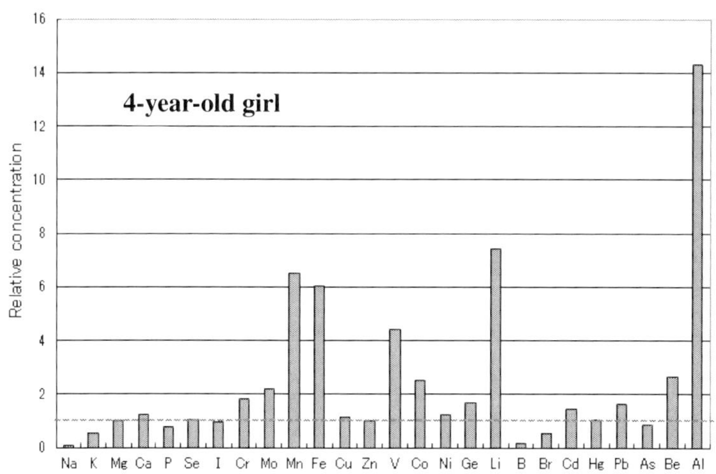

Figure 4. Mineral imbalance profile of autistic child with high aluminium burden. Another typical metallomics profile of 4-year-old girl with autism is shown, exhibiting simultaneous high burdens with aluminium (53.7 ppm), manganese (702 ppb), iron (37.0 ppm) and lithium (12.2 ppb) [22]. Each bar represents the relative concentration of the respective trace element in her scalp hair specimen. The dotted horizontal line at 1.0 represents the reference control level of each trace element.

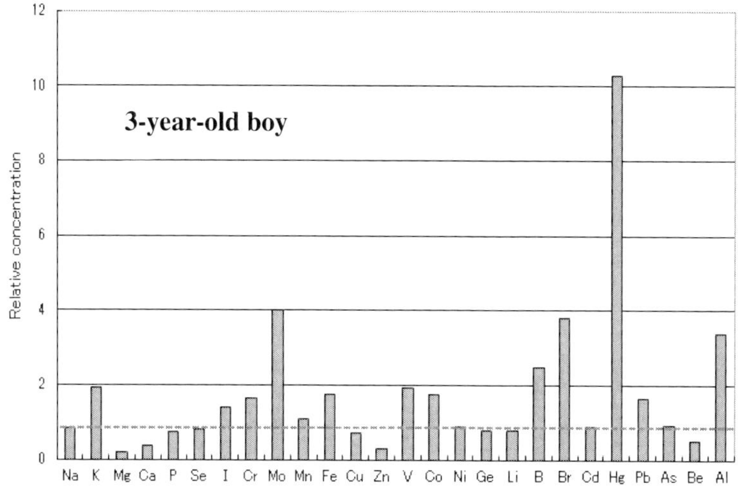

Figure 5. Mineral imbalance profile of autistic child with high mercury burden. Other typical metallomics profile of a 3-year-old boy with autism is shown, exhibiting a high burden with mercury of over 10-fold level (40.1 ppm) [22]. Each bar represents the relative concentration of the respective trace element in his scalp hair specimen. The dotted horizontal line at 1.0 represents the reference control level of each trace element.

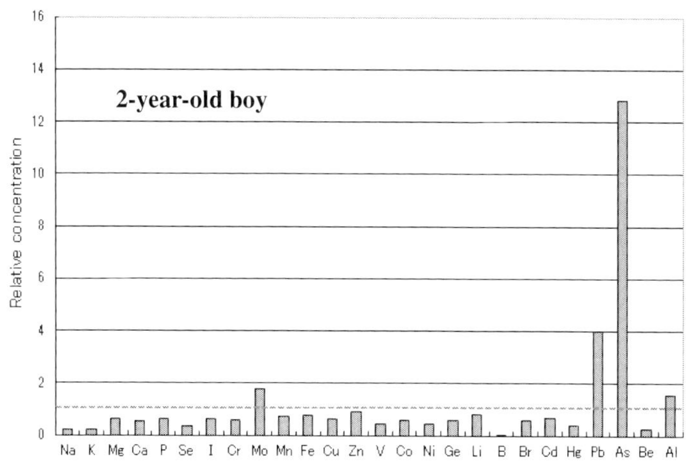

Figure 6. Mineral imbalance profile of autistic child with high arsenic burden. Other typical metallomics profile of a 2-year-old boy with autism is shown, exhibiting a high burden with arsenic of over 12-fold level (655 ppb) [22]. Each bar represents the relative concentration of the respective trace element in his scalp hair specimen. The dotted horizontal line at 1.0 represents the reference control level of each trace element.

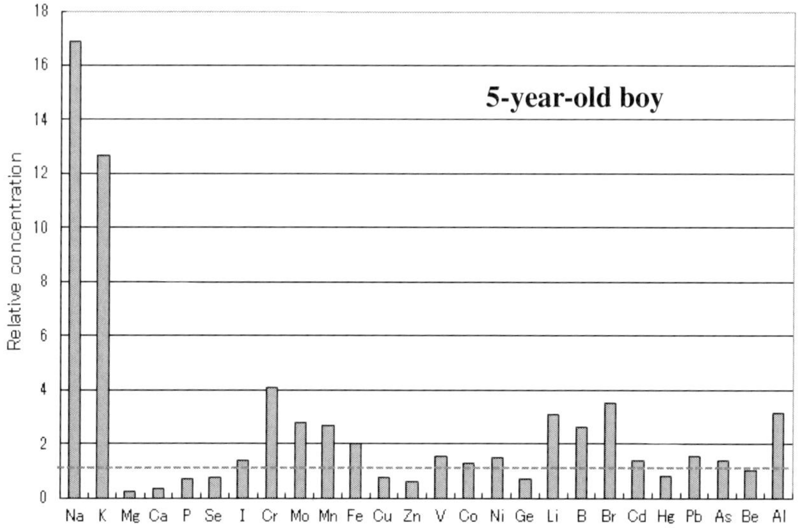

Figure 7. Mineral imbalance profile of autistic child with high sodium/potassium levels. Other typical metallomics profile of 5-year-old boy with autism is shown, exhibiting simultaneous high burdens with sodium (335 ppm) and potassium (210 ppm) [22]. Each bar represents the relative concentration of the respective trace element in his scalp hair specimen. The dotted horizontal line at 1.0 represents the reference control level of each trace element.

3.5. Infantile Time Window in Neurodevelopment and for Therapy

The age at final diagnosis of autism spectrum disorders ranges from 3 to 6 years, although most cases of autism are diagnosed by the age of three and as early as 14 months [35]. In facts, zinc deficiency was detected in many of the infantile patients in the first 3 years of life (Figure 1), and high toxic metal burdens were also detected in the autistic subjects, especially in the younger children [19-22,36]. Thus, for treatment/prevention of autism spectrum disorders, its early screening and estimation is necessary and it is desirable to early check any metabolic and mineral disorders for the infants and children with autistic symptoms, though there are serious limitations of diagnosis of the younger children. It should be considered that the pathogenesis of neurodevelopment disorders might start in prenatal phase and is progressive within the time window for exact diagnosis.

3.6. Autism-Related Genes and Epigenetic Alteration by Mineral Disorders

Zinc is a structural component of zinc-finger proteins and a transcriptional regulator, and influences some candidate genes reported to be associated with the development of autism, such as MTF1 (metal-responsive transcription factor 1), metallothionein, ZnT5 (zinc transporter 5), COMMD1 (COMM domain-containing protein 1), ERK1 (extracellular signal-regulated kinase 1), TrkB (tyrosine-related kinase B), SHANK2 and SHANK3 (SH3 and multiple ankyrin repeat domains), and also ProSAP1 and ProSAP2 (proline-rich synapse-associated protein), or themselves are involved in zinc signalling and homeostasis [37-41]. Thus, zinc deficiency observed in the autistic subjects (Figure 1 and 3) might induce critical epigenetic alterations to provide a central mechanism of gene/environment interaction to interfere with neuronal maturation during early development [20-22,40-42].

Magnesium deficiency has been reported to cause changes in the methylation of several genes, leading to affect their expression and function, embryonic development and metabolic disturbances connected to several diseases [43,44].

In addition, high toxic metal burdens detected in the autistic patients (Figure 3-6) seem contribute to the mechanism of gene/environment interaction, because cadmium, arsenic, lead and mercury have been reported to be candidate factors that induce epigenetic alterations such as DNA methylation and histone modifications [11-15,41,45] and neurodevelopmental disorders [16,21,22,40-42]. One case-control study of 196 families with at least two ASD children has found some association between ASD and SNPs in the divalent metal ion transporter SLC11A3 and metal regulatory transcription factor 1 (MTF1) [46]. SLC11A3 is involved in the intracellular transport of heavy metals of iron, lead, cadmium and nickel, and MTF1 is important in the activation of metallothionein after exposure to heavy metals: both factors seem role to reduce heavy metal toxicity.

It remains to be clarified what epigenetic and pathogenesis mechanisms do relate to various mineral imbalances observed in autistic patients (Figure 3-7).

4. Discussion

Zinc ion functions as the active site in more than 300 kinds of enzymes and about 10% in the total gene-coded proteins have been known to have zinc-finger sequences [31,32], emphasizing the physiological importance of this trace element and the epigenetic roles of zinc deficiency in the pathogenesis of genetic diseases. In brain hippocampus, zinc is co-stored with glutamate in pre-synaptic vesicles in the excitatory neuron terminal, is released from them and controls the activity of excitatory glutamate receptors on post-synaptic excitable membrane [33,34]. Thus, zinc deficiency was reported to affect learning, memory and neurogenesis and associate with neurological disorders and neurodegenerative diseases [47-50].

Recently we found that many infants with autistic disorders are suffered from marginal to severe zinc deficiency, suggesting considerable relationship of infantile zinc deficiency with autism [20]. Furthermore, we demonstrated that infantile autistic children are liable to deficiency in magnesium and calcium next to zinc, but not in the other essential metals [21,22]. These findings suggest that autistic infants and probably infants themselves have a characteristic liable and susceptible to zinc- and magnesium-deficiency, because larger amounts of the trace elements (per kg body weight) are needed for the neurodevelopment and growth.

There are numerous studies with the same theme reporting nutritional status and mineral deficiencies in autistic children [51-55], although the restricted age (over 4-year-old) and small number of children and restricted minerals were examined and so their conclusions were not consistent, and the critical environmental factors remained to be established. In our metallomics study for the 1,967 autistic children aged 0-15 year-old, we have demonstrated not only the critical, epigenetic factors (zinc- and magnesium-deficiency and high burdens of aluminium, cadmium, lead and so on) but also the presence of another critical term factor, "infantile time window" in neurodevelopment and probably for therapy [20-22].

Recently, Kurita et al. [56] reported that zinc deficiency in utero induces fetal epigenetic alterations of histone modifications in metallothionein 2 promoter region having metal responsive elements in 1-day-old and 5-week-old mice, of which pregnant mother were fed low zinc diet from gestation day 8 until delivery.

Gebremedhin et al. [57] reported that compared to pregnant women aged 15-24 years, those aged 25-34 and 35-49 years had 1.57 (95%CL: 1.04-2.34) and 2.18 (95%CL: 1.25-3.63) times higher risk of zinc deficiency, respectively. Their study demonstrated that old age pregnancy is negatively associated to zinc status, probably suggesting that one of the origins of the high incidence rate of infantile zinc deficiency may be higher age pregnancy of their mothers.

Arnold et al. [58] reported that mean serum zinc levels were significantly lower in both autism and ADHD groups, and that serum zinc level correlated inversely with parent- and teacher-rated inattention in ADHD children. Furthermore, zinc treatment was reported significantly superior to placebo in reducing symptoms of hyperactivity, impulsivity and impaired socialization in ADHD patients [59,60]. Other preliminary human study showed that many children with ADHD have lower zinc concentration in comparison to healthy children and zinc supplement as an adjunct to methylphenidate has favourable effects in the treatment of ADHD children, pointing to the possible association of zinc deficiency and ADHD pathophysiology [61].

Kozielec et al. [62] have reported that in hyperactive 116 children with ADHD, magnesium deficiency was found in the 95 % of the subjects, most frequently in hair (77.6%), next in red-blood cells (58.6 %) and in blood serum (33.6 %). Furthermore, they reported that in the group of ADHD children given 6 months of magnesium supplementation, a significant decrease of hyperactivity and increase in hair magnesium contents has been achieved [63]. Mousain-Bosc et al. [64] also reported that 52 hyper-excitable children have low intra-erythrocyte magnesium levels with normal serum magnesium values, and that magnesium/vitamin B6 supplementation can restore the erythrocyte magnesium levels to normal and improve their abnormal behaviours. They also reported that thirty-three children with clinical symptoms of pervasive developmental disorder (PDD) or autism exhibit significantly lower red blood cell magnesium values, and that the combination therapy with magnesium/vitamin B6 for 6 months improved significantly PDD symptoms in 23/33 children ($p < 0.0001$) with concomitant increases in intra-erythrocyte magnesium values [65].

These findings suggest that infantile zinc- and magnesium-deficiency play epigenetically principal roles as environment factors in the pathogenesis of neurodevelopment disorders such as autism spectrum disorders and ADHD, and that there is a critical term "infantile time window" in neurodevelopment and probably for treatment and prevention of these genetic disorders.

Recently, dietary restriction-induced zinc deficiency has been reported to up-regulate intestinal zinc-importer (ZIP4) and induce the increase in ZIP4 protein located to the plasma membrane of enterocytes [66,67]. This adoptive response to zinc deficiency is known to lead to increasing in the risk of high-uptake of toxic metals such as cadmium and lead [68]. Thus, infants with zinc deficiency are liable to increased risk of absorbing high amount of toxic metals and retaining them in their bodies, as shown in Figure 2, which demonstrates a high significant inverse relationship between zinc and lead level. These findings suggest that the increased toxic metal burdens attendant on zinc deficiency may also epigenetically contribute to the pathogenesis of these diseases.

Deficiency in magnesium/calcium is reported to enhance the toxic effects of lead (Pb) on cognitive and behavioural development in children [69]. A significant inverse relationship between dietary calcium intake and blood lead concentrations has been found in 3,000 American children examined as part of NHANES II [70]. Elevated blood lead levels are found in some children diagnosed with autism and associated with the development of ADHD [70,71].

About 250,000 children in the U.S. A. have high blood lead (Pb) levels over the current level of concern of 10μg/dL [72], despite significant progresses over the past half century in reducing child lead poisoning rates [73]. This number is likely to double or more as the U.S. Centers for Disease Control and Prevention (CDC) considers the recommendation to lower the Level of Concern from 10μg/dL to 5μg/dL [74]. This major change in national policy is based on a large and growing body of evidence showing that even single-digit blood Pb levels have significant impacts on Intelligence Quotients, Attention Deficit Hyperactivity Disorder (ADHD) risks, cardiovascular disease, and kidney function [75-79].

The most common lead exposure pathway for children are ingestion or inhalation of lead-bearing road dusts, whether in the household or outdoor environment [80-82], and its most common sources are fossil fuels, asphalt and paints (lead chromate or lead carbonate) [82-84]. In addition, maternal cigarette smoking has been reported to be associated with lower zinc and higher cadmium and lead concentrations in their neonates [85]. These toxic metals accumulated in the maternal bone tissues are co-transferred with calcium to foetal and newborn bodies through activated bone-resorption during pregnancy and lactation [85-88]. In fact, a recent birth cohort study for new-borns in Nepal shows that the motor cluster score was inversely associated with the cord blood levels of lead and arsenic, suggesting that high exposures to Pb and As during the prenatal period may induce retardation during in-utero neurodevelopment [89].

Eklund and Oskarsson [90] reported that soy-based formulas contain approximately six times more cadmium than cow's milk formulas, and cereal-based formulas have 4-21 times higher levels. Thus, the dietary intake of the toxic metal in the children feeding on infant formulas and weaning foods may be higher in comparison with breast milk-fed infants.

For mercury and arsenic, the maximum burden levels of 9.3- and 33.5-fold of the reference level may also epigenetically play any pathogenic roles in the respective autistic individuals, even though their incidence rates were 2.8 % or less. It is expected to demonstrate that these mineral disorders induce the epigenetic deficits in autism-related genes, such as eIF4E-dependent system [91] and other candidate genes. In near future, we hope it will be clarified what type of metallomics profiles does associate with what disorder in various behaviour/neurological deficits in autism spectrum disorders ?

In summary, this review demonstrates that many of autistic infants have been suffered from various mineral imbalances such as marginal to severe zinc- and magnesium-deficiency and/or high toxic metal burdens of aluminium, cadmium, lead and so on. These findings suggest that infantile mineral imbalances, due to their epigenetic adverse effects, probably play principal roles in the pathogenesis of diverse autism spectrum disorders. Furthermore, these infantile autistic patients with mineral imbalances in their bodies could respond to a novel evidence-based nutritional approach which supplements deficient nutrients and detoxifies accumulated toxic metals. This evidence-based nutritional approach may yield a new pathway into early screening/assessment and treatment/prevention of infantile patients with autism spectrum disorders including the suspects. Well-controlled intervention studies for this novel nutritional therapy are desired to establish the epigenetic roles of infantile mineral disorders in the pathogenesis of neurodevelopment disorders and to develop an early assessment and therapy of neurodevelopment disorders such as autism spectrum disorders, ADHD and the suspects.

Conclusion

This chapter demonstrates that many of infantile patients with autism spectrum disorders are suffered from marginal to severe zinc- and magnesium-deficiency and/or high toxic metal burdens of aluminium, cadmium, lead and so on, suggesting that these mineral imbalances in bodies may play principal, epigenetic roles as environment factors in the pathogenesis of the neurodevelopment disorders and that there is a critical term “infantile time window” in neurodevelopment and for their therapy. In near future, an innovative introduction of novel clinical tests such as metabolomics and metallomics analysis is desired for early assessment and intervention/ treatment of autistic children.

Acknowledgments

The author appreciates the autistic subjects and their relatives for collaboration to this study. The author thanks T. Tsutsui for his supports to this study and colleagues for their technical contributions to trace element analysis.

Competing Financial Interests

The author declares no competing financial interests.

References

[1] Weintraub, K. Autism counts. *Nature* 479, 22-24 (2011).

[2] Pinto, D. *et al.* Functional impact of global rare copy number variation in autism spectrum disorders. *Nature* 466, 368-372 (2010).

[3] Chakrabarti, S. & Fombonne, E. Pervasive developmental disorders in preschool children: confirmation of high prevalence. *Am. J. Psychiatry* 162, 1133-1141 (2005).

[4] Bailey, A. *et al.* Autism as a strongly genetic disorder: evidence from a British twin study. *Psychol. Med.* 25, 63-77 (1995).

[5] Marshall, C.R. *et al.* Structural variation of chromosomes in autism spectrum disorder. *Am. J. Hum. Genet.* 82, 477-488 (2008).

[6] Kim, S.J. et al. A quantitative association study of SLC25A12 and restricted repetitive behavior traits in autism spectrum disorders. *Mol. Autism* 2 (1), 8 (2011).

[7] Murdoch, J.D. & State, M.W. Recent developments in the genetics of autism spectrum disorders. *Curr. Opin. Genet. Dev.* (2013).

[8] Hughes, V. Autism: Complex disorder. *Nature* 491, S2-S3 (2012).

[9] Dufault, R. *et al.* Mercury exposure, nutritional deficiencies and metabolic disruption may affect learning in children. *Behav. Brain Funct.* 5, 44-58 (2009).

[10] O'Rahilly S. Human genetics illuminates the paths to metabolic disease. *Nature* 462, 307-314 (2009).

[11] Jin, Y.H. *et al.* Cadmium is a mutagen that acts by inhibiting mismatch repair. *Nat. Genet.* 34, 239-241 (2003).

[12] Takiguchi, M., Achanzar, W.E., Qu, W., Li, G. & Waalkes, M.P. Effects of cadmium on DNA-(cytosine-5) methyltransferase activity and DNA methylation status during cadmium-induced cellular transformation. *Exp. Cell Res.* 286, 355-365 (2003).

[13] Arita, A. & Costa, M. Epigenetics in metal carcinogenesis: nickel, arsenic, chromium and cadmium. *Metallomics* 1, 222-228 (2009).

[14] Perera, F. & Herbstman, J. Prenatal environmental exposure, epigenetics, and disease. *Reprod. Toxicol.* 31, 363-373 (2011).

[15] Jakovcevski, M. & Akbarian, S. Epigenetic mechanisms in neurological disease. *Nat. Med.* 18, 1194-1204 (2012).

[16] Ciesielski, T. et al. Cadmium exposure and neurodevelopmental outcomes in U.S. children. *Environ. Health Persp.* 120, 758-763 (2012).

[17] Yasuda, H., Yonashiro, T., Yoshida, K., Ishii, T. & Tsutsui T. High toxic metal levels in scalp hair of infants and children. *Biomed. Res. Trace Elem.* 16, 39-45 (2005).

[18] Yasuda, H., Yoshida, K., Segawa, M., Tokuda, R., Yasuda, Y. & Tsutsui, T. High accumulation of aluminium in hairs of infants and children. *Biomed. Res. Trace Elem.* 19, 57-62 (2008).

[19] Yasuda, H., Yoshida, K., Yasuda, Y. & Tsutsui, T. Two age-related accumulation profiles of toxic metals. *Cur. Aging Sci.* 5, 105-111 (2012).

[20] Yasuda, H., Yoshida, K., Yasuda, Y. & Tsutsui, T. Infantile zinc deficiency: Association with autism spectrum disorders. *Sci. Rep.* 1, srep00129 (2011).

[21] Yasuda, H., Yasuda, Y. & Tsutsui, T. Estimation of autistic children by metallomics analysis. *Sci. Rep.* 3, srep01199 (2013).

[22] Yasuda, H. & Tsutsui, T. Assessment of infantile mineral imbalances in autism spectrum disorders (ASDs). *Int. J. Environ. Res. Public Health* 10, 6027-6043 (2013).

[23] Rodushkin, I. & Axelsson, M.D. Application of double focusing sector field ICP-MS for multi elemental characterization of human hair and nails. Part I. Analytical methodology. *Sci. Total Environ.* 250, 83-100 (2000).

[24] Goulle, J.P. *et al.* Metal and metalloid multi-elementary ICP-MS validation in whole blood, plasma, urine and hair: Reference values. *Forens. Sci. Intern.* 153, 39-44 (2005).

[25] Wang, C.T., Chang, W.T., Zeng, W.F. & Lin, C.H. Concentrations of calcium, copper, iron, magnesium, potassium, sodium and zinc in adult

female hair with different body mass indexes in Taiwan. *Clin. Chem. Lab. Med.*43, 389-393 (2005).

[26] Yasuda, H., Yonashiro, T., Yoshida, K., Ishii, T. & Tsutsui, T. Mineral imbalance in children with autistic disorders. *Biomed. Res. Trace Elem.* 16, 285-291 (2005).

[27] Munakata, M. *et al.* A preliminary analysis of trace elements in the scalp hair of patients with severe motor disabilities receiving enteral nutrition., *Brain Development* 28, 521-525 (2006).

[28] Yasuda, H., Yonashiro, T., Yoshida, K., Ishii, T. & Tsutsui, T. Relationship between body mass index and minerals in male Japanese adults. *Biomed. Res. Trace Elem.* 17, 316-321 (2006).

[29] Yasuda, H. *et al.* Metallomics study using hair mineral analysis and multiple logistic regression analysis: relationship between cancer and minerals. *Environ. Health Prev. Med.* 14, 261-266 (2009).

[30] Ochi, A. *et al.* Elemental concentrations in scalp hair, nutritional status and health-related quality of life in haemodialysis patients. *Therap. Apheresis Dialysis* 16, 127-133 (2012).

[31] Prasad, A.S. Impact of the discovery of human zinc deficiency on health. *J. Am. Coll. Nutr.* 28, 257-265 (2009).

[32] Fukada, T., Yamasaki, S., Nishida, K., Murakami, M. & Hirano, T. Zinc homeostasis and signalling in health and diseases: Zinc signalling. *J. Biol. Inorg. Chem.* 16, 1123-1134 (2011).

[33] Takeda, A. Movement of zinc and its functional significance in the brain. *Brain Res. Rev.* 34, 137-148 (2000).

[34] Takeda, A., Nakamura, M., Fujii, H. & Tamano, H. Synaptic Zn(2+) homeostasis and its significance. *Metallomics* 5, 417-423 (2013).

[35] Landa, R.J. Diagnosis of autism spectrum disorders in the first 3 years of life. *Nat. Clin. Pract. Neurol.* 4, 138-147 (2008).

[36] Yasuda, H. & Tsutsui, T. Infants and elders are liable to zinc deficiency (submitted).

[37] Huang, Y.Z., Pan, E., Xiong, Z.,Q. & McNamara, J.O. Zinc-mediated transactivation of TrkB potentiates the hippocampal mossy fiber-CA3 pyramidal synapse. *Neuron* 57, 546-558 (2008).

[38] O'Roak, B.J. et al. Exome sequencing in sporadic autism spectrum disorders identifies severe de novo mutations. *Nat. Genet.* 43, 585-589 (2011).

[39] Sanders, S.J. et al. De novo mutations revealed by whole exome sequencing are strongly associated with autism. *Nature* 485, 237-241 (2012).

[40] Grabrucker, A.M. Environmental factors in autism. *Front. Psych.* 3, 1-13 (2013).

[41] Dufault, R., Lukiw, W.J., Crider, R., Schnoll, R., Wallinga, D. & Deth, R. A macroepigenetic approach to identify factors responsible for the autism epidemic in the United States. *Clin. Epigen.* 4 (1), 6 (2012).

[42] Wessels, I. Epigenetics and Metal Deficiencies. *Cur. Nut. Rep.* 3, 196-203 (2014).

[43] Takaya, J., Iharada, A., Okihana, H. & Kaneko, K. Magnesium deficiency in pregnant rats alters methylation of specific cytosines in the hepatic hydroxysteroid dehydrogenase-2 promoter of the offspring. *Epigenetics* 6, 573-578 (2011).

[44] Komiya, Y., Su, L.T., Chen, H.C., Habas, R. & Runneis, L.W. Magnesium and embryonic development. Magnes. Res. 27, 1-8 (2014).

[45] Ray, P.D., Yosim, A. & Fry, R.C. Incorporating epigenetic data into the risk assessment process for the toxic metals arsenic, cadmium, chromium, lead, and mercury: strategies and challenges. *Front Genet.* 5, 201 (2014).

[46] Serajee, F.J., Nabi, R., Zhong, H. & Huq, M. Polymorphisms in xenobiotic metabolism genes and autism. *J. Child Neurol.* 19, 413-417 (2004).

[47] Arnold, L.E. & DiSilvestro, R.A. Zinc in attention-deficit/hyperactivity disorder. *J. Child Adolesc. Psychopharmacol.* 15, 619-627 (2005).

[48] DiGirolamo, A.M. & Raminez-Zea, M. Role of zinc in maternal and child mental health. *Am. J. Clin. Nutr.* 89 (suppl), 940S-945S (2009).

[49] Scheplyagina, L. A. Impact of the mother's zinc deficiency on the woman's and new-borns health status. *J. Trace Elem. Med. Biol.* 19, 29-35 (2005).

[50] Plum, L.M., Rink, L. & Haase, H. The essential toxin: Impact of zinc on human health. *Intern. J. Environ. Res. Public Health* 7, 1342-1365 (2010).

[51] Yorbik, O., Akay, C., Sayal, A., Cansever, A., Sohmen, T. & Cavdar, A. O. Zinc status in autistic children. *J. Trace Elem. Exp. Med.* 17, 101-107 (2004).

[52] Fido, A. & Al-Saad, S. Toxic trace elements in the hair of children with autism. *Autism* 9, 290-298 (2005).

[53] Adams, J. B., Holloway, C. E., George F. & Quig, D. Analyses of toxic metals and essential minerals in the hair of Arizona children with autism and associated conditions, and their mothers. *Biol. Trace Elem. Res.* 110, 193-209 (2006).

[54] Faber, S., Zinn, G. M., Kern J. C. & Kingston, H. M. The plasma zinc/serum copper ratio as a biomarker in children with autism spectrum disorders. *Biomarkers*, 14, 171-180 (2009).

[55] Lakshmi Priya, M. D. & Geetha, A. Level of trace elements (copper, zinc, magnesium and selenium) and toxic elements (lead and mercury) in the hair and nail of children with autism. *Biol. Trace Elem. Res.* 142, 148-158 (2011).

[56] Kurita, H., Ohsako, S., Hashimoto, S., Yoshinaga, J. & Tohyama, C. Prenatal zinc deficiency-dependent epigenetic alterations of mouse metallothionein-2 gene. *J. Nutr. Biochem.* 24, 256-266 (2013).

[57] Gebremedhin, S., Enquselassie, F. & Umeta, M. Prevalence of prenatal zinc deficiency and its association with socio-demographic, dietary and health care related factors in Rural Sidama, Southern Ethiopia: A cross-sectional study. *BMC Public Health* 11, 898-907 (2011).

[58] Arnold, L. E. *et al.* Serum zinc correlates with parent- and teacher- rated inattention in children with attention-deficit/hyperactivity disorder. *J. Child Adoles. Psychopharmacol.* 15, 628-636 (2005).

[59] Yorbik, O., Ozdag, M.F., Olgun, A., Senol, M.G., Bek, S. & Akman, S. Potential effects of zinc on information processing in boys with attention deficit hyper-activity disorder. *Progr. Neuropsychopharmacol. Biol. Psychiatry*, 32, 662-667 (2008).

[60] DiGirolamo, A.M. *et al.* Randomized trial of the effect of zinc supplementation on the mental health of school-age children in Guatemala. *Am. J. Clin. Nutr.* 92, 1241-1250 (2010).

[61] Akhondzadeh, S., Mohammadi, M.R. & Khademi, M. Zinc sulfate as an adjunct to methylphenidate for the treatment of attention deficit hyperactivity disorder in children: a double blind and randomised trial [ISRCTN64132371]. *BMC Psychiatry*, 4, 9-14 (2004).

[62] Kozielec, T. & Starobrat-Hermelin, B. Assessment of magnesium levels in children with attention deficit hyperactivity disorder (ADHD). *Magnes. Res.* 10, 143-148 (1997).

[63] Starobrat-Hermelin, B. & Kozielec, T. The effects of magnesium physiological supplementation on hyperactivity in children with attention deficit hyperactivity disorder (ADHD). Positive response to magnesium oral loading test. *Magnes. Res.* 10, 149-156 (1997).

[64] Mousain-Bose, M., Roche, M., Rapin, J. & Bali, J.P. Magnesium VitB6 intake reduces central nervous system hyperexcitability in children. *J. Am. Coll. Nutr.* 23, 545S-548S (2004).

[65] Mousain-Bose, M., Roche, M., Polge, A., Pradal-Prat, D., Rapin, J. & Bali, J.P. Improvement of neurobehavioral disorders in children supplemented with magnesium-vitanin B6 II. Pervasive developmental disorder-autism. *Magnes. Res.* 19, 53-62 (2006).

[66] Dufner-Beattie, J., Kuo, Y.M., Gitschier, J. & Andrews, G.K. The adaptive response to dietary zinc in mice involves the differential cellular localization and zinc regulation of the zinc transporters ZIP4 and ZIP5. *J. Biol. Chem.* 279, 49082-49090 (2004).

[67] Lichten, L.A. & Cousins, R.J. Mammalian zinc transporters: nutritional and physiologic regulation. *Ann. Rev. Nutr.* 29, 153-176 (2009).

[68] Goyer, R.A. Toxic and essential metal interactions. *Ann. Rev. Nutr.* 17, 37-50 (1997).

[69] Mahaffey, K.R., Gartside, P.S. & Glueck, C.J. Blood lead levels and dietary calcium intake in 1 to 11 year-old children: the second national health and nutrition examination survey, 1976 to 1980. *Pediatrics* 78, 257-262 (1986).

[70] Shannon, M. & Graef, J.W. Lead intoxication in children with pervasive developmental disorders. *J. Toxicol. Clin. Toxicol.* 34, 177-181 (1996).

[71] Eubig, P.A., Agular, A. & Schantz, S.L. Lead and PCBs as risk factors for attention deficit/hyperactivity disorder. *Environ. Health Perspect.* 118, 1654-1667 (2010).

[72] Centers for Disease Control and Prevention (CDC). *CDC National Surveillance Data (1997-2009), National Centers for Environmental Health* 2012. Available on line: http://www.cdc.gov/nceh/lead/data/national.htm.

[73] Jones, R.L.; Homa, D.M.; Meyer, P.A.; Brody, D.J.; Caldwell, K.L.; Pirkle, J.L.; Brown, M.J. Trends in blood lead levels and blood testing among US children aged 1 to 5 years, 1988-2004. *Pediatrics* 123, 376-385 (2009).

[74] Advisory Committee on Childhood Lead Poisoning Prevention, of the Centers for Disease Control and Prevention (ACCLPP). Low Level Lead Exposure Harms Children: A renewed Call for Primary Prevention: Report to the CDCP; ACCLPP: Atlanta, GA, USA, 2012; pp. 1-54.

[75] Needleman, H.L.; Schell, A.; Bellinger, D.; Leviton, A.; Allred, E.N. The long-term effects of exposure to low doses of lead in childhood. An 11-year follow up report. *N. Engl. J. Med.* 322, 83-88 (1990).

[76] Binns, H.J.; Campbell, C.; Brown, M.J. Interpreting and managing blood lead levels of less than 10 micro g/dL in children and reducing childhood exposure to lead: Recommendations of the Centers for Disease Control

and Prevention Advisory Committee on Childhood Lead Poisoning Prevention. *Pediatrics* 120, e1285-e1298 (2007).

[77] Bellinger, D.C. Lead neurotoxicity and socioeconomic status: Conceptual and analytical issues. *Neurotoxicology* 29, 828-832 (2008).

[78] Gump, B.B.; Stewart, P.; Reihman, J.; Lonky, E.; Darvill, T.; Parsons, P.J; Granger, D.A. Low-level prenatal and postnatal blood lead (Pb) exposure and adrenocortical responses to acute stress in children. *Environ. Health Perspect.* 116, 249-255 (2008).

[79] Nigg, J.T.; Knottnerus, G.M.; Martel, M.M.; Nikoas, M.; Cavanagh, V.; Karmaus, W.; Rappley, M.D. Low blood lead levels associated with clinically diagnosed attention-deficit/hyperactivity disorder and mediated by weak cognitive control. *Biol. Psychiatry* 63, 325-331 (2008).

[80] Dixon, S.L.; Gaitens, J.M.; Jacobs, D.E.; Strauss, W.; Nagaraja, L., Pivetz, T.: Wilson, J.W.; Ashley, P.J. Exposure of U.S. children to residential dust lead, 1999-2004: II. The contribution of lead-contaminated dust to children's blood lead levels. *Environ. Health Perspect.* 117, 468-474 (2009).

[81] American Academy of Pediatrics. Lead exposure in children: Prevention, detection, and management: Statement of policy reaffirmation. *Psychiatry* 123, 1421-1422 (2009).

[82] Deocampo, D.M.; Reed, P.J.; Kalenuik, A.P. Road dust lead (Pb) in two neighbourhoods of urban Atlanta, (GA, USA). *Int. J. Environ. Res. Public Health* 9, 2020-2030 (2012).

[83] Hall, G.; Tinklenberg, J. Determination of Ti, Zn, and Pb in lead-based house paints by EDXRF. *J. Anal. Atom. Spectr.* 18, 775-778 (2003).

[84] Lewis, P.A. Inorganic colored pigments. In *Paint and Coating Testing Manual*, 14th ed.; Koleske, J.V., Ed.; ASTM; West Conshohocken, PA, USA, 1995; pp. 1-950.

[85] Symanski, E. & Hertz-Picciotto, I. Blood lead levels in relation to menopause, smoking, and pregnancy history. *Am. J. Epidemiol.* 141, 1047-1058 (1995).

[86] Razagui, I.B. & Ghribi, I. Maternal and neonatal scalp hair concentrations of zinc, cadmium, and lead: relationship to some lifestyle factors. *Biol. Trace Elem. Res.* 106, 1-28 (2005).

[87] Gulson, B.L., Jameson, C.W., Mahaffey, K.R., Mizon, K.J., Korsch, M.J. & Vimpani, G. Pregnancy increases mobilization of lead from maternal skeleton. *J. Lab. Clin. Med.* 130, 51-62 (1997).

[88] Sanders, A.P. *et al.* Towards prenatal biomonitoring in North Carolina: Assessing arsenic, cadmium, mercury and lead levels in pregnant women. *PLoS ONE* 7, e31354 (2012).
[89] Parajuli, R.P., Fujiwara, T., Umezaki, M. & Watanabe, C. Association of cord blood levels of lead, arsenic, and zinc with neurodevelopmental indicators in newborns: A birth cohort study in Chitwan Valley, Nepal. *Environ. Res.*10, 509-519 (2012).
[90] Eklund, G. & Oskarsson, A. Exposure of cadmium from infant formulas and weaning foods. *Food Addit. Contam.* 16, 509-519 (1999).
[91] Gkogkas, C.G. et al. Autism-related deficits via dysregulated eIF4E-dependent translational control. *Nature* 493, 371-377 (2013).

In: Autism Spectrum Disorders
Editor: Arlene Valdez
ISBN: 978-1-63482-547-4

Chapter 3

Student and Family Involvement in Transition Planning: Promising Practices and Student Outcomes

David Hagner[1*] and Alan Kurtz[2]
[1]University of New Hampshire, Institute on Disability
[2]University of Maine
Center on Community Inclusion and Disability Studies

Studies of transition outcomes have consistently documented disappointing employment and community living outcomes for individuals with an autism spectrum disorder (ASD) (Billstedt, Gillberg, & Gillberg, 2011; Cederlund, Hagberg, Billstedt, Gillberg, & Gillberg, 2008; Howlin, 2013; Liptak, Kennedy, & Dosa, 2011; Targett & Wehman, 2009; Taylor & Mailick, 2014). To some extent, the poor transition outcomes for individuals on the autism spectrum can be attributed to poor quality transition planning (Schall, 2009). Many planning processes are driven more by a concern for compliance with regulations than by a strong desire to ensure students leave high school prepared to achieve an expansive vision of adult life (Edmundson & Cain, 2003).

* Email: david.hagner@unh.edu.

A key feature of high quality transition planning is the active involvement of the individual and their family in the process (Cobb & Alwell, 2009; Landmark, Song, & Dalun, 2010). Families play a major role in socializing children to the norms and values of adulthood, but the process is also to some degree collaborative, as emerging adults also socialize their parents, and parents socialize each other (Roest, Dubas, & Gerris, 2009). Thus, goals are set and decisions made jointly by students and their parents (Young, Marshall, Dornene, Graham, Logan, Zaidman, Mart, & Lee, 2008). Transition planning is most effective when it takes advantage of and builds upon these efforts, rather than supplanting them with a professionally-driven approach in which youth and families are only marginally involved. Individuals with disabilities and their families are in the best position to know what they need (Deguara, Jelasi, Micallef, & Callus, 2012).

One approach to facilitating active involvement, Family-Centered Transition Planning (FCTP), has demonstrated significantly improved outcomes over traditional transition planning. The approach uses a combination of group family training sessions and a series of individual planning meetings and assistance from a planning facilitator to work on plan implementation, including career exploration activities, work experiences, and coordinating plans with other services.

In this chapter, we present the FCTP approach and the results that have been achieved by students and families. We will also devote specific attention to the central role that changes in student and parent expectations play in the process, both as results of and drivers of the transition planning process, and outline a theoretical account of the key elements that lead to empowered action by students and families. Finally, we will report current efforts to replicate and sustain the FCTP model.

Transition Planning for Individuals on the Autism Spectrum

Unemployment and underemployment are common among individuals across the spectrum (Howlin, Goode, Hutton, & Rutter, 2004; Targett & Wehman, 2009). Youth in the U.S. with ASD have the lowest rate of employment among all disability groups (Roux, Shattuck, Cooper, et al., 2013). Estimates of employment rates have varied from 25% to 50% (Hendricks, 2010; Holwerda, van der Klink, Groothoff, & Brouwer, 2012).

Researchers analyzing National Longitudinal Transition Study-2 data have found that just over 50% of youth with ASD had worked at some time during their first six years following high school (Chiang, Cheung, Li, & Tsai, 2013; Eaves & Ho, 2008; Liptak et al., 2011; Roux et al., 2013; Shattuck, Narendorf et al., 2012), and that the rate of full-time employment never exceeded 15% (Wei, Wagner, Hudson, Yu, & Shattuck, 2014). Youth with both ASD and intellectual disability were least likely to be employed (Gray, Keating, et al., 2014; Hendricks, 2010; Holwerda, et al., 2012).

Individuals with ASD tend to be disproportionately employed in menial jobs involving assembly, sorting, stuffing and cleaning (Newman, Wagner, Knokey, et al., 2011). Youth with ASD also work for significantly lower wages and more limited hours than youth with other disabilities (Roux et al. 2013; Chiang et al., 2013). Eaves and Ho (2008) found that youth with ASD averaged only five hours of paid work each week.

Poor employment outcomes are far from inevitable. A number of studies have demonstrated that youth with ASD, including individuals with significant social, cognitive, communication, and behavioral support needs, can work with appropriate supports and planning (Targett & Smith, 2009; Targett & Wehman, 2009).

Employment planning is especially important given the multiple benefits of employment for youth with ASD. Most view their work experiences positively (Migliore & Zalewska, 2012). Research also demonstrates that youth with ASD not only benefit financially from working (Cimera & Burgess, 2011), but are likely to experience a reduction in both autism symptoms and maladaptive behavior and an increase in skills related to activities of daily living (Taylor, Smith & Mailick, 2014).

Researchers have also documented poor community living and educational outcomes for youth with ASD. Individuals with ASD seldom reside in community living situations in which they can demonstrate the level of independence typical in our culture (Billstedt, Gillberg & Gillberg, 2011; Howlin et al., 2004; Targett & Smith, 2009). Eaves and Ho (2008) found that 56% of young adults with ASD were living with their families and 35% were living in supported living arrangements.

Young adults with ASD have been found to have fewer friends and smaller social networks than their peers without disabilities (Cederlund et al., 2008). Only one in three reported having a close friend (Eaves & Ho, 2008). Using a large nationally representative sample, Liptak et al. (2011) found that youth with ASD experienced serious social isolation and that they tended to become increasingly isolated over time. Over 50% had not spent time with friends in the previous year and almost two thirds had not spoken to a friend on the phone in that time. Contrary to popular conceptions, research suggests that most individuals with ASD desire friendships and social interaction and that they become increasingly important as they move into adolescence and adult life (Carrington, Templeton, & Papinczak, 2003; Locke, Ishijima, Kasari, & London, 2010; McGovern & Sigman, 2005).

Increasingly postsecondary education of some kind is considered to be a viable option for many youth with ASD (Briel & Getzel, 2009; Holmes & Chaffee, 2007). However, individuals with ASD need intensive supports and careful planning to succeed in postsecondary education (Adreon & Durocher, 2007; Briel & Getzel, 2009; Roberts, 2010; VanBergeijk, Klin & Volkmar, 2008). But an analysis of student IEPs found that only 23% of youth with ASD had goals related to attending college (Migliore & Lugas, 2011), suggesting that transition planning is often inadequate in this area.

There is a clear link between student and family participation in transition planning and positive adult outcomes (DeFur, 2003; Landmark, Song, & Dalun, 2010; Shogren, et al., 2007; Test et al., 2009). Nevertheless, planning often fails to adequately involve the student and family (Chambers et al., 2004; Hetherington et al., 2010; Schall, 2009). Shogren and Plotner (2012) reported that compared to those with other disabilities, youth with ASD participate less in their transition planning meetings, are less likely to take a leadership role in the meetings, and are less likely to participate in identifying transition goals. These investigators also found that about 35% of parents of youth with ASD express dissatisfaction with their participation in the transition process, despite the fact that the transition to adulthood is one of two periods in the lives of individuals with ASD when families are likely to need the most intensive supports – the other being when ASD is first diagnosed (Russa, Matthews, & Owen-DeSchryver, 2014).

One reason for the neglect of family perspectives may be that professionals tend to assume that they are already sufficiently familiar with their viewpoints (Bourke-Taylor, Howie & Law, 2010). As Green (2007) noted, such professional assumptions are often either mistaken or are oversimplifications.

A second explanation may be connected to the complexity of adult system state and federal programs and funding streams (Chambers, Hughes, & Carter, 2004; Schall & Wehman, 2009). Adult service systems are often overlapping, fragmented and uncoordinated (Hetherington et al., 2010; Waisman Center, 2009; Test, Smith, & Carter, 2014; Wittenburg, Golden, & Fishman, 2002), with no single point of entry (Revell & Miller, 2009). Faced with this complexity, parents find it difficult to engage as informed participants in transition planning (Briel & Getzel, 2009; Certo et al., 2003; Holmes & Chaffee, 2007; Holmes & Shore, 2005; Waisman Center, 2009).

Tehee, Honna, and Hevey (2009) found that a lack of adequate information and education was a significant source of stress for the parents of individuals with ASD, especially in connection with a "concern for the future" (p. 40). In addition, they found that parents' access to information and education varied with the age of the child, with the families of adolescents (age 15-18) reporting that they received significantly less information than the parents of other age groups.

In addition to causing stress, lack of information about adult options and supports can lead to low parental expectations (Carter, Trainor, Ditchman, Swedeen, & Owens, 2009). Ivey (2004) found that parents of youth with autism often had low expectations that their children would ultimately hold a job, could remain safe from harm, live independently, or have a network of friends. These low expectations can result in youth being excluded from employment and other community experiences (Carter, Trainor, Cakiroglu, Swedeen, & Owens, 2009), and thus set up a vicious cycle of low achievement followed by even lower expectations. Thus it is not surprising that Chiang et al. (2013) found that improved employment outcomes for youth with ASD are associated with higher parent expectations.

Family-Centered Transition Planning

Family-Centered Transition Planning (FCTP) assists an individual with a disability, together with friends, family members, professionals and others, to work collaboratively to plan for life beyond high school based on individual strengths, needs, and preferences. The model is based on person-centered planning, an approach that has been found to be effective in helping people with disabilities achieve employment, obtain social support, and participate more actively in their communities (Holburn, Jacobson, Schwartz, Flory, & Vietze, 2004; Robertson et al., 2006). Person-centered planning strategies can also lead to increased participation in IEPs during the transition period (Test et al., 2004), because issues and requests are developed and discussed in advance of the formal meeting (Ruppar & Gaffney, 2011). Person-centered planning has been found to be especially helpful to individuals with ASD as they explore post school options for employment and community life (Schall, 2009; Targett & Wehman, 2009).

The Three-Component Process

FCTP is an outgrowth of person-centered planning but focuses on the entire family as decision makers and as the focus of support (Kim & Yurnbull, 2004). The approach is a service package consisting of three components provided over an 8-10 month period: Parent training, person-centered planning, and career exploration assistance.

Parent training. For the first component, parents receive group training in post-school options, resources, and planning techniques. There are six training topics, which can be scheduled either as six late afternoon/evening sessions – one topic per session, or as three full day sessions, covering two topics per day. We found that the three-day option – one Saturday per month for three months – works best if some families are traveling some distance. The six training topics are as follows:

1. Orientation to Planning: The important role families can play in creating a meaningful life and support network for their son/daughter after leaving high school. This session also includes an orientation to the adult service system, focusing on issues and challenges impacting transition outcomes and individualized/consumer-directed services.
2. Assuming Personal Power: Strategies for assuming a leadership role in the planning process. This session offers examples and activities to help participants understand group dynamics, brainstorming, and the role of creativity in group planning, to avoid the pitfalls to empowered action, and to understand the importance of building an effective personal support team.
3. Tools for Planning: Graphic organizers useful for creating flip charts for group planning that draw out important information about an individual's strengths, learning styles and support needs. This information builds a foundation for developing meaningful goals for work, home, and social opportunities.
4. Designing Opportunities & Supports: Practical approaches for approaching decision-makers and resource people to and creating opportunities, including information about a broad range of options for custom-designing supports and services.
5. Using Resources Wisely: Strategies for creatively combining and maximizing resources to cover the cost of supports and services. This session provides information about key funding sources and

programs, such as Medicaid, Social Security, and Vocational Rehabilitation.

6. Getting To Action: Following a summary of the training, participants to identify next steps for creating a meaningful routine and support network for their son/daughter after leaving high school.

The training sessions include refreshments and meals, and participants receive a binder with materials for each session. The sessions are taught by two trainers, a parent who has gone through the transition process and an individual knowledgeable about programs and funding. A group size of between eight and twelve participants is ideal, both for sharing and peer support and from a cost point of view. At least one parent or caregiver must attend each session, and both parents are welcome.

Person-centered planning. After parent training has begun, a facilitator is matched to each family for facilitating a series of person-centered planning meetings to enable each student to plan transition goals. Planning meetings are held at the convenience of each student and family. Other family members, friends, and community resource people often participate in one or more meetings. Facilitators assist each student to prepare for maximum participation.

Facilitators must be skilled in transition planning and in facilitating groups, and they must be free of any connections to services that the individual might receive or be interested in, in order to serve only the student and family without any conflicting interests. Planning begins any time after the start of parent training sessions, but not prior to the first parent session. Between six and eight meetings are held, until a post-school plan is developed. Table 1 provides a general Service Timeline for planning sessions.

The planning process is highly individualized, and adaptations of the typical person-centered planning process are sometimes employed to meet the specific needs of individuals on the autism spectrum who may have communication difficulties or experience anxiety in group meetings. Strategies facilitating participation include: (1) individualized preparation for meetings, (2) informal activities to build rapport between the planning facilitator and the youth, (3) flexible meeting designs, (4) distance attendance, and (5) support for alternative means of communication (Hagner, Kurtz, May, & Cloutier, 2014). For example, one student was uncomfortable speaking in his meetings. He and his project mentor (an adult with ASD who served on the project team) created a PowerPoint presentation outlining his interests and vision for a future life.

Table 1. Family Centered Transition Planning General Service Timeline

Family Training	Family-Centered Planning	Outputs
Obtain family commitment to session schedule.	Enrollment Meeting/Interview Enrollment paperwork Establish purpose for planning Complete Vocational Decision-Making Inventory	
Session 1*		
	Facilitator / family match; Role clarifications with families, youth, facilitator	
	1st Meeting Meeting purpose – purpose of tools ("maps") Set groundrules Timeline *Relationships* Extending invitations - Who else to include in the planning Set next meeting agenda	Digital photos & brief summary of meeting to attendees, coordinator, funder(s).
Session 2*		
	2nd Meeting *Preferences* *Learning styles*, what works/ doesn't work *Communication*/ relationships/ supervision style *Strengths*/ accomplishments/ skills	Digital photos & brief summary of meeting to attendees, coordinator, funder(s).
	3rd Meeting (Optional tools) *Visions* *Current Routine* *Places* Structured brainstorm Assignments/ research – participant homework assignments	Digital photos & brief summary of meeting to attendees, coordinator, funder(s). Mid-term report to funders
	4th Meeting *Goals* *Strategies* *Action Plan*	Digital photos & brief summary of meeting to attendees, coordinator, funder(s).

Family Training	Family-Centered Planning	Outputs
Session 3*		
	5Th - 6th Meeting Finalize plan Identify support needs Brainstorm available resources Research options Educate family/ team about options, and talking to others about goals (internship, volunteering, apprenticeship) Identify who is making what commitments	Digital photos & brief summary of meeting to attendees, coordinator, funder(s).
	7th Meeting Create draft budget for long term goals Specify language/ job descriptions for any potential long term support people Next Steps - who needs copies of the plan Partnership for transition implementation	Final report, if required by finder(s), including goals and plan for achieving goals: Who, what, when, where.

*Sessions can be earlier than this in the process, but not later.

The mentor read the slides but the student clarified or elaborated when necessary. He also answered questions at the end. Another student participated in meetings from his bedroom by Skype. A variety of strategies can be used to support a person's communication in meetings. One youth indicated whether he agreed with what was being said by giving a "thumbs up" or "thumbs down" sign. Another used an augmentative and alternative communication device to communicate in meetings. One youth expressed his dissatisfaction with his participation in the previous meeting, complaining that he was "out-talked." In the next meeting his school tutor sat next to him and helped him compose notes. When each note was finished, the tutor announced that the student had something to add, and the student read the note aloud.

Career exploration. For this third FCTP component, facilitators provide assistance and encouragement in exploring emerging ideas and possibilities, including career exploration and work experiences linked to the evolving planning process. Typical activities include informational interviews, job shadowing experiences, online or in-person investigation of post secondary options, and paid or unpaid part-time or summer work.

Facilitators also assist students and families to incorporate elements of student plans into student IEPs and if necessary assist in applying to adult service agencies. Because the goal is for students and families to identify what they want for their future, and then to advocate for themselves and work towards it, the role of a facilitator is not to serve as a direct advocate for a family with funders. A facilitator may attend an IEP or similar meeting and may assist families to communicate a request, or participate in brainstorming and prioritizing, but does not "take sides" as a direct advocate for or against a party to a disagreement. Plan implementation assistance includes helping students and families understand what they can expect and what expenses are allowable by various funding sources, and what consumer rights and complaint procedures apply. But facilitators also take care to explain the reality that funding is limited and that unreasonable requests often backfire, and that a spirit of compromise and willingness to prioritize what is most important and not insist on getting everything is most effective. Facilitators also help students and families look creatively at multiple sources of assistance, including natural and informal supports. This can include looking at the kinds of assistance and support parents typically provide to their teenage and young adult children without disabilities – such as paying fees and tuition and providing transportation – and encouraging them to apply a similar standard to a child with a disability.

Illustrative Examples

Perhaps the best way to get a sense of what FCTP works in the real world is through examples that illustrate the process. The following stories, one from Maine and one from New Hampshire, are representative.

Jeff. Jeff is a young man whose ability to communicate verbally is limited. For most of his life he has shown a strong interest in cooking. When asked where he would like to gain some experience cooking, he named several local fast-food restaurants. After some discussion with his team he agreed that an internship at a local college known nationally for the quality of its food services might be a better option. Team members helped arrange a successful internship at the college. After graduation Jeff found a paid job working six hours a week as a baker at a retirement community, and he also volunteers for the local school district in the cafeteria.

Jeff's mother also believed that he could learn to drive and that he should get his driver's license. A Vocational Rehabilitation Counselor felt that he was not a good candidate to drive and would not provide funding for training to get his license. Jeff's mother decided that, in her words, she "would not take 'no' for an answer." This approach was something she learned though the parent training. She found a private driving instructor who agreed to teach Jeff to drive and to provide the training again for free if he did not pass his driver's test. He succeeded on the first try, and was able to drive to his Senior Prom.

Dominick. Dominick is a talented musician who expressed an interest in pursuing a college degree in music and a music career. A team was developed to help create a plan to achieve his goals. Dominick interviewed his orchestra instructor, and was advised to take private music lessons and join marching band and chorus. A meeting with his school team revealed that he was lacking a foreign language and a math class that would be required for college admission. Dominick joined the marching band and took chorus, and arranged to alter his school schedule to include a new math class, but adding a foreign language class was not feasible, and he found that he could not afford private music lessons. His planning team found creative ways to overcome these obstacles. He arranged to barter his services by teaching beginner lessons in return for the music lessons he needed. To substitute for a foreign language, Dominick noted on his college application that he was fluent in American Sign Language (because he has a brother with a hearing impairment). This was acceptable to the college, and Dominick was admitted to and currently attends his first choice college. And after high school he was hired for a paid position playing oboe in a community band.

Student Outcomes

Family-Centered Transition Planning began with a two-year demonstration project in New Hampshire and Maine, followed by a three-year period that focused on gradually shifting implementation responsibility to community service providers and extending the scope of the project to a third state. Pre and post quantitative data were collected during this time on variables highly correlated with post-school success. Additional analyses of this data examined the impact of joint planning and the impact of plan timing within the transition process. Employment and postsecondary education outcome data were then collected through a follow-up study of the participants in the original demonstration after they had completed high school.

Demonstration Project Outcomes

To conduct the initial demonstration project, project staff contacted School Special Education and Transition Coordinators and the Transition Counselors in Vocational Rehabilitation regional offices in southern Maine and a five-county region of New Hampshire, provided information about the program. These individuals were asked to distribute the information and project contact information to youth on the autism spectrum between the ages of 16 – 24 and their families. Those indicating an interest in the project were provided information about the program and both the youth and one family member was enrolled upon consent. Diagnosis on the autism spectrum was verified through the Autism Diagnostic Observation Schedule (ADOS).

Pre and post data were collected on expectations for the future, vocational maturity/decision-making, and self-determination. Expectation data consisted of the expectations section of the National Longitudinal Transition Survey II (Wagner, Newman, Cameto, Levine, & Garza, 2006), consisting of eight questions rating expectations from 1 (definitely won't) to 4 (definitely will). Four questions concerned postsecondary education and four concerned independence (residential independence, financial independence, employment, driver's license). Total scores ranged from 8 – 32.

Vocational decision-making was assessed using the Vocational Decision-Making Interview - Revised (VDMI-R). This instrument was designed for use with individuals with disabilities and follows a structured interview format with 54 questions about jobs and the job selection process. Strong reliability and validity have been reported for the VDMI-R (Tiffany, 2004).

Self-Determination was measured using the ARC Self-Determination Scale (adolescent version). This self-report measure was designed for use with individuals with cognitive disabilities (Wehmeyer & Kelchner, 1995), and measures four domains of self-determination: Autonomy, self-regulation, psychological empowerment, and self-realization.

In the first year of the project, enrolled participants were randomly assigned to a year one and a year two group. The year one group received services immediately, and the year two group began one year later. This allowed the year two group to serve as a control group to test the effectiveness of the FCTP intervention. Data were collected on both groups at enrollment and one year later, prior to the start of services for the year two group. After completing FCTP, participants in the year one group reported significantly higher levels of self-determination, career decision-making, and higher expectations for the future, and their parents also reported significantly higher expectations for the future than participants in the control group (Hagner, Kurtz, Cloutier, Arakelian, Brucker & May, 2012).

After the year two group received services, plans were made to gradually shift implementation responsibility from university grant-funded staff to local community service provider organizations, and to extend the project to a third state. Community service provider organizations in New Hampshire and Maine were selected and trained to implement FCTP, and additional groups of students and families in each state were enrolled. A few other changes were made at this point as well. We switched from using the ARC Self-Determination scale to the Self-Determination Scale developed by the American Institutes of Research (AIR) because it provides subscales that distinguish between self-determination opportunities and self-determination skills (Wolman, Campeau, DuBois, Mithaug & Stolarski, 1994). And we accepted a confirmation of a diagnosis on the autism spectrum through school record rather than administering the ADOS.

By using community service providers, we intended to transfer implementation of FCTP to existing service and funding organizations that would, over time, replace the need for a grant-funded University project and ensure sustainabilty (Fixsen, Naoom, Blasé, Friedman & Wallace, 2005) when grant funding ended. In year three, a community service provider in ME and NH were responsible for recruitment and selection of participants and overall coordination, while project staff continued to provide parent training and planning facilitation. In year four, the project continued to provide parent training, and responsibility for facilitation was shared between community service providers and project staff. We also extended FCTP services at this point to a third demonstration site, the Los Angeles area.

The project provided technical assistance and continued to train planning facilitators through a credit-bearing graduate course offered at the University of New Hampshire, *Methods, Models and Tools for Person-centered Planning*. Also in year four, local funding sources were required to cover community provider facilitation costs. To accomplish this, each community service provider organization established a fee for service rate and cost structure, and student referrals had to be accompanied by an assurance of funding from one of three sources: A school, a vocational rehabilitation office, or a developmental service office. The goal was to establish a seamless transition process as recommended by Certo and Luecking (2011) by combining funding from all three sources, so that the resulting cost for each funding source would be small. However, having three different organizations each with its own eligibility criteria and procedures work together proved to be a formidable challenge. Combined funding remains a work in progress, and for year four, it was typically easiest for one or the other funding source to pay the full service fee.

In all, 58 youth and 58 family members were enrolled, and six participants dropped out before completing the program, so that data is available on 52 students and families who completed FCTP. We examined the impact of FCTP for this group on transition variables, supplemented by analyses of expectations across participants and the impact of plan timing.

Impact on transition variables. Pre-post data on student and parent expectations and vocational decision-making were analyzed using repeated measures t-tests. We found that students initially had higher expectations (mean = 26.3) than their parents (mean = 22.2), and that following FCTP there were statistically significant increases in both student and parent expectations to means of 28.4 and 25.1, respectively. One-tailed t-tests showed that both of these increases were statistically significant (Hagner & Kurtz, in review). And an increase in student vocational decision-making from a mean of 22.38 to 26.68 was also statistically significant.

When broken down into two cohorts, those served with exclusively university implementation in years one and two and those served with joint implementation by university and community provider personnel in years three and four, both cohorts experienced statistically significant increases in parent expectations and highly significant increases in vocational decision-making, but there was only a slight, non-significant increase in student expectations in the second cohort (Hagner & Kurtz, in review).

Self-determination data collected in years one and two using the ARC Self-Determination Scale showed a statistically significant increase from 59.7 to 73.9 following FCTP, whereas in the control group, the change over that time period from 62.3 to 67.1 was not statistically significant, and was likely due to a combination of typical transition programming and student maturation. And in years three and four, using the AIR Self-determination Scale, we also found a statistically significant increase in self-determination as measured by students and parents, from a mean of 69.8 to a mean of 75.7. However, when the self-determination opportunities and skills subscales were tested separately, parent responses indicated significant increases in both opportunities and skills; but student responses indicated a significant increase in self-determination skills but only a small, non-significant increase in self-determination opportunities. It may be that students were becoming more aware of their roles as active agents directing their own futures.

Expectations and collaborative planning. The impact of FCTP on student and parent expectations is particularly important because of the strong role they play in influencing opportunities and on eventual post-school achievement (Ivey, 2004; Wong & Heriot, 2007). A brief summary of research on expectations will set the stage for an analysis of collaborative planning.

The future expectations of parents of youth with ASD have been consistently found to be low. Ivey (2004) found that on a scale measuring the likelihood of a positive outcome as 1 (least likely) to 5 (most likely), the mean rankings of parents were: financial security, 4.04; obtaining highest education possible and having a job, 3.92, and living independently, 3.36. When parents were asked how important these outcomes were for their children, importance was rated significantly higher than likelihood.

Other studies have reported similar results. In Wong and Heriot's (2007) investigation of the hope and despair held by the parents of children with autism, they found that 80% had low hope and high despair for their child. It should be noted that Wong and Heriot (2007) included the parents of children with childhood dementia in their sample. Although estimates vary, intellectual disability frequently co-occurs with ASD (Lecavalier, Snow, & Norris, 2011). Kraemer and Blacher (2001) found that parent ideal views of positive vocational outcomes for their children with severe intellectual disabilities often included employment in independent or supported settings, but that these views were inconsistent with their realistic views, which included employment in more restrictive settings. And parental expectations for their child with ASD's participation in postsecondary education are tempered by their expectation that there are significant obstacles to success (Camarena & Sarigiani, 2009).

Transitioning youth with disabilities tend to have higher expectations for themselves than their parents have. Powers, Geenen, and Powers (2009) found that while youth and their parents agreed on the most important transition goals, youth viewed themselves as more prepared to achieve them than their parents.

Several investigators have examined the degree to which youth and parent expectations change over time during adolescence. Powers, Geenen, and Powers (2009) found no difference in the views of parents and students about transition goals and services as the youth grow older. However, Clare and Garnier (2000) found that parent goals for their adolescent children were adjusted upwards to align more with the child's current functioning than with the parents' earlier goals, suggesting that parental expectations are subject to change over time.

Another focus of investigation has been on the impact of family relationships on expectations. We have seen that parents play a major role in socializing children to the norms and values of adulthood, but also that emerging adults socialize their parents, and parents socialize one another (Roest, Dubas, & Gerris, 2009). This lends itself to a collaborative process of goal-setting and decision-making (Young, Marshall, Dornene, Graham, Logan, Zaidman, Mart, & Lee, 2008). Roest, Dubas and Gerris (2009) found that this collaborative process is enhanced in families with a more positive family climate. Germeijs and Verscheren (2009) also found that the quality of parent/child interactions affect a child's transition planning. Perceived security with a child's mother predicted a higher awareness of the need for planning and higher levels of exploratory behavior, both self and environmental, for adolescents.

Scales and Benson (2011) also focused on the quality of child/parent interactions as a significant factor influencing readiness for adulthood. They theorized that three youth assets or strengths – the identification and development of a passion for a self-identified interest, supportive relationships and opportunities for empowerment – promote developmental experiences that foster academic, psychological, and behavioral well-being. However, they found that only 9% of young adolescents report that they possess high levels of all 3 of these strengths, and 28% report none of them (Scales & Benson, 2011). These authors recommended interventions that improve the degree to which adolescents have caring supportive relationships and enhance their sense of empowerment.

Family-Centered Transition Planning focuses on the family as a unit, supports positive parent-child interactions, and promotes joint exploration of youth interests and passions, as recommended by Scales and Benson (2011). Thus, we investigated whether student and parent expectations become more convergent following FCTP, indicating that both parties moved in the direction of more collaborative planning.

Correlation coefficients for student and parent expectations before and after FCTP showed that the pre-intervention correlation of 0.35 more than doubled, to 0.78, following FCTP. This greater convergence in expectations on the part of students and parents suggests that FCTP helped students and families to view transition issues in more similar ways. This is an important finding because, as Young et al. (2008) pointed out, joint planning and problem-solving may be more effective when the parties to the process approach the situation from similar perspectives.

Plan timing. The timing of transition planning may also influence outcomes. Hetherington, Durant-Jones, Johnson, Nolan, Smith, Taylor-Brown and Tuttle (2010) noted that planning often comes too late to affect outcomes to a great degree, and thus, earlier introduction of transition panning might be expected to have a more pronounced effect on expectations. Cimera, Burgess and Wiley (2013) compared Rehabilitation Services Administration outcome data for individuals with autism spectrum disorders from states where transition services beginning at age 14 with those where planning begins at age 16. Individuals in the earlier planning states were more likely to be employed, received higher wages, and their services cost less than those in the later planning states.

Does it make a difference whether FCTP takes place earlier or later in the transition process? Students entered the demonstration project at different points in their transition years, and their schools varied in graduation policies. This created a natural experiment whereby the timing of family-centered transition planning differed across students. Planning for each family could be ordered as occurring (a) before the next-to-last year of high school ($n = 12$), (b) during the next to last year of high school ($n = 11$), (c) during the last year of high school ($n = 14$), or (d) during the year after leaving high school ($n = 7$). To investigate whether timing matters, nonparametric Kruskal-Wallis statistics were calculated using overall change in expectations as the dependent variable across the four timing categories. There was no significant difference either for students ($H = 3.12$, $p = 0.37$) or parents ($H = 2.69$, $p = 0.44$) associated with the timing of planning in relation to changes in expectations (Hagner & Kurtz, in review). There was also no significant difference in vocational decision-making ($H = 3.42$, $p = .33$) across the four groups. It may be that the quality of planning is more important than its timing.

Follow-Up Study

A follow-up study collected employment and education outcome data on the participants in the first two years of the FCTP demonstration project. These participants, who had been by that time out of high school between two and three years, were contacted by telephone or email. Of those responding, 89% were employed, 75% in paid jobs and 14% in unpaid volunteer positions. (Some of those with paid jobs had additional unpaid jobs as well). Work hours averaged 13.7 per week, and those with paid jobs had an average hourly wage of $9.06. In addition, 50% of the respondents were enrolled in postsecondary education; 17% in four-year programs, 28% in two-year programs, and 6% in special college campus programs for individuals with disabilities. These results far exceed those obtained in national studies of this population (Newman, et al., 2011; Shattuck, Narendor, Cooper, Sterzine, Wagner, & Taylor, 2012) and other transition demonstration reports (e.g., Taylor & Seltzer, 2010).

Parent Perspectives on Transition Involvement

We have seen that families have a major role in to play in facilitating the transition to adult life, and for that reason FCTP was designed as an intervention for families as well as for their children on the autism spectrum. Thus it is important to understand the process from the family's point of view.

We conducted semi-structured interviews with a sub-sample of families in the demonstration project. Qualitative analysis of interviews can offer the opportunity to explore the process in more depth, and perhaps help us understand some of the relationships among the complex factors at work in transition planning. Families were selected for interviews whose children had at least one more year of high school ahead of them at the time they completed the FCTP process, so that we could examine how FCTP affected the relationship between the family, the student, and the school.

Five families in New Hampshire and four in Maine were interviewed between 8 and 10 months following the end of project services. One interview in each state was by telephone, due to difficulties making scheduling arrangements, and the remaining seven interviews were conducted in-person in family homes. Interviews were guided by a series of open-ended questions, as follows: (a) What are your and your child's goals for after s/he finishes high school, and how clear are you about these goals? (b) What steps are you taking or planning to take to reach these goals? (c) How confident are you that these goals will be reached? (d) Do you have any worries about reaching your goals? (e) In what way(s) did your participation in the FCTP project affect the goals that you and your child are working towards, or change the way you planned? (f) What was most helpful and least helpful about the project for you? (g) Did you make any requests of the school based on the planning you did through the project? What was their response? (h) Did you make any requests of any other agency or organization? What was their response? (i) Has your view of the strengths and potential of your child changed at all since you have been involved with the project, and if so, how? (j) Do you have any recommendations for other families going through the transition process?

The children of the families interviewed were between 18 and 21 years old when the interviews took place. They included eight men and one woman. All nine students lived with their natural families. Each of the nine children of the families interviewed attended their neighborhood public school. Two attended the same school, and each of the remaining seven attended a different school.

One interview was with a student's grandmother, who was his primary caregiver, and one interview was conducted with a student's father and mother together. The remaining seven interviews were with the student's mother. The interview data were organized into coding categories based on content similarity by two interviewers independently coding the full set of interview transcriptions. The two interviewers combined their coding categories into a single set of themes and study findings under each theme. These themes and findings then served as the basis for constructing a tentative theoretical account of the key elements of family involvement in transition.

Family Interview Findings

The interview findings can be summarized under five major themes: (a) family experiences with transition planning, (b) student participation in planning, (c) awareness of student strengths and potential, (d) access to transition resources, and (e) responses to parent advocacy.

Transition experiences. A common theme across all of the interviews was the value of educational and informational sessions for helping parents understand post-school options, prioritize what should be done when, and parcel out transition responsibilities into manageable tasks. As one family member put it, this "helped us focus."

Interviewees consistently reported that receiving training on transition options changed their perceptions about what was possible for their child in adult life. In some cases learning about a wider array of options provided parents with a sense of relief. As one parent explained: "It was nice to know that he did not have to go to day hab. We didn't want that and he wouldn't want that."

Training sessions also resulted in family members viewing their children differently. As one interviewee indicated,

> (The training) was extremely helpful in helping us bring down the barriers of what she can't do, and focusing on what she can do. I am certain that, going into the program, we were more aware of her deficits than we were of her capabilities.

Families also appreciated the opportunity the group training provided to interact with other family members engaged in similar experiences. They also found person-centered planning sessions helpful. One interviewee felt that the planning sessions built upon the foundation created by the group training sessions, saying that it "sort of reinforced what we learned in a more personal way." Another family member reported that: "My dining room looked like flip chart heaven. But it was good. (The facilitator) made us think of a lot of different options."

Interviewees also viewed as helpful the way planning facilitators modeled perseverance in working towards goals and following through on plans. As one interviewee put it,

> It's one thing to sit for a couple of Saturdays and be told to think outside the box. It's quite another for (the facilitator) to never say die. Just unbelievable modeling, and perseverance, and tenacity to show that if you keep looking for stuff, surprisingly enough, you'll find it.

Families appreciated meetings in the family's home, scheduled at the family's convenience. The emphasis on involving other supportive people in planning also helped give families an expanded vision of the network of people could be called upon for support. One interviewee noted that "You will often, as parents, think you are kind of alone in this game. It was helpful to see the list on the wall – the list of people that can help you get to places, go in different directions." Another family member discussed her realization that there were other people could help them support their son's transition:

> My tendency is to overprotect him and to think that nobody else will do as good as me in knowing what's right for him. It was eye opening to know that there are people out there who do want to help him. I don't have to protect him from the whole world, just some of it. It isn't just me who is going to get him out there. I am limiting him by making it just me. I need to allow other people to help him.

All of the respondents wished that ideally a similar service could be available throughout the entire transition process, but with one exception families reported continued progress in working towards post-school employment or postsecondary education goals. One family out of the nine interviewed reported that they had made almost no progress since services had discontinued, and that they wanted more hands-on assistance with filling out applications for services and meeting with adult services about eligibility.

Student participation in planning. Families reported that the planning process had been growth-enhancing for their children. For many, this manifested itself in an increased ability of their child to advocate for himself or herself. One interviewee reported that her son spoke at his IEP meeting for the first time as a result of his participation in planning: "Last week he answered questions at his IEP. He never did that before. He was able to talk about what he wanted." Another interviewee noted that her son made an appointment to see his guidance counselor about dropping a course he disliked; something she believed that he would never have done before. Another was impressed that her son was able to conduct interviews of potential employment service staff members, and select the one he liked best. One parent explained that her daughter had "learned through this process to become her own self-advocate."

Several families reported that their children experienced a degree of discomfort or anxiety in connection with participating in planning meetings. One parent explained that her daughter had become more aware of "who she is and what her challenges are. This was anxiety-provoking." However, even when students felt uncomfortable or anxious during planning meetings, the difficulty was described as minor, and could even be described as a positive experience. As another parent noted, "Nobody grows up without a little bit of tension."

Awareness of student strengths and potential. Several parents began the transition process feeling, as one interviewee put it, that they "had trouble imagining" a positive future for their child. At the time of the interviews, families reported that they had become more clearly aware of their child's strengths and potential. The following statement by a mother of a student who was planning on going away to college in a few months is representative of these comments:

> I had her living at home and not going to college. It just wasn't on my radar as a possibility for her. But between her advocating for herself and us kind of really realizing her strengths, we went in a totally different direction than we would have.

Student accomplishments mentioned by families in connection with receiving planning assistance included obtaining a driver's license, and, in one case, driving to the Senior Prom with his date. A number of students had acquired meaningful job skills or had done well in college classes. One parent was amazed with the cooking skills acquired by her son through a culinary training program, noting that, "When he makes things at home now, everything is all chopped up to be all the same size. It's a work of art."

Another parent spoke of being impressed by the level of self-awareness indicated by a poem written by his child:

> Father: He has written what I thought was a very interesting poem. What was that called?
>
> Mother: "What I Would Do in 100 Days."
>
> Father: Yes, It was very poignant. It brought tears to my eyes. I mean just to hear his interpretation of his ability, and what he would do, and how he would go about doing it, and what he would get out of it. I thought that was really good. I mean, for lack of a better word, this is a kid who showed insight.

Access to transition resources. We have noted that parent involvement in planning helped them to think more creatively about accessing resources for transition, and "look at broader ranges of possibilities than I had in the past", as one interviewee put it. Noteworthy in this regard was the wide variety of informal and typical resources that students accessed for entry into adult life. These included friends, relatives, other community members, clubs and teams, and universally available technology such as "i-pads." For example, one student felt that it was stigmatizing for a paraprofessional to accompany him throughout his school day, so the family requested that he no longer be assigned a paraprofessional. But, as this family related,

> He was missing out on completing a lot of assignments, because nobody reminded him that he had the assignment. So we taught him to pull that i-pad out, which everyone thinks is cool, and it also allows him to do assignments on his own.

As another example, a planning group brainstormed the personal connections they had with business owners in their town, and scheduled meetings with their contacts to develop a job for their child.

Formal disability service resources were also used in nontraditional ways. For example, one student arranged for his high school to provide transportation to a local community college during his last year in school so he could try out a college class. This same student also arranged to work on an independent project called "A History of Me" for high school history credit.

A striking example of creative thinking occurred when one family realized that in order for their son to receive the college financial aid he needed, he had to be 18 years old, and he would not turn 18 until several weeks into the first semester. The family engaged an attorney to obtain court approval for emancipation of their child as an adult prior to his 18th birthday, to allow him to qualify. This family reported that their training and experience with planning encouraged them to approach transition obstacles like this in a creative way.

Responses to parent advocacy. Participation in Family-Centered Transition Planning allowed students and families to develop a vision for a positive future and become more clearly aware of what was needed to achieve that vision. This resulted in several instances where requests for specific services were made to schools and adult disability organizations.

Families received mixed reception to requests made to schools. Many special education programs were willing to entertain individualized requests. One school, for example, agreed to contribute towards the tuition cost of a summer arts institute for a student interested in pursuing a career in the arts. The family paid the remaining tuition. Other requests that were granted included assigning a staff person to develop a work experience opportunity and providing transportation so that a student could participate in an after-school club. But not all requests were granted. In three cases, in three different schools, families requested an additional year of school to allow their child to work on transition goals, arguing that even though enough credits would be technically earned for graduation, arrangements would not yet be in place for a smooth transition. One request was granted and two were denied. One family indicated that there was no follow-through from the school and said of the family-centered plan they developed, "The school wouldn't even look at it."

The experiences of families in this project with adult service organizations were uniformly negative. In one case, an organization providing employment experiences used a level of one-to-one job coaching to support their son on a work experience that the family felt was unnecessary. And in all six cases where families had attempted to receive assistance from the state Vocational Rehabilitation system, their experiences were described in negative terms. One family described the experience as "abysmal", and another reported that "Voc. Rehab. has never shown up for meetings. They have not done anything." The process was described as slow, frustrating, and unproductive for their children. One parent voiced her frustration:

> We've been working with the same [vocational rehabilitation] person now since the school year started, and she just this morning brought another version of a proposal to get him into a program to get him a job. It's like, "Will you stop writing proposals and just get him a job!"

A Theory of Family Empowerment

A number of core similarities were evident in the accounts related by parents of the process leading to the articulation of a positive future for their transition-aged child with ASD and the ability to identify and persevere in advocating for resources to implement the plan. These core similarities can serve as the basis for constructing a tentative theoretical account of the key elements that lead to this type of empowered action.

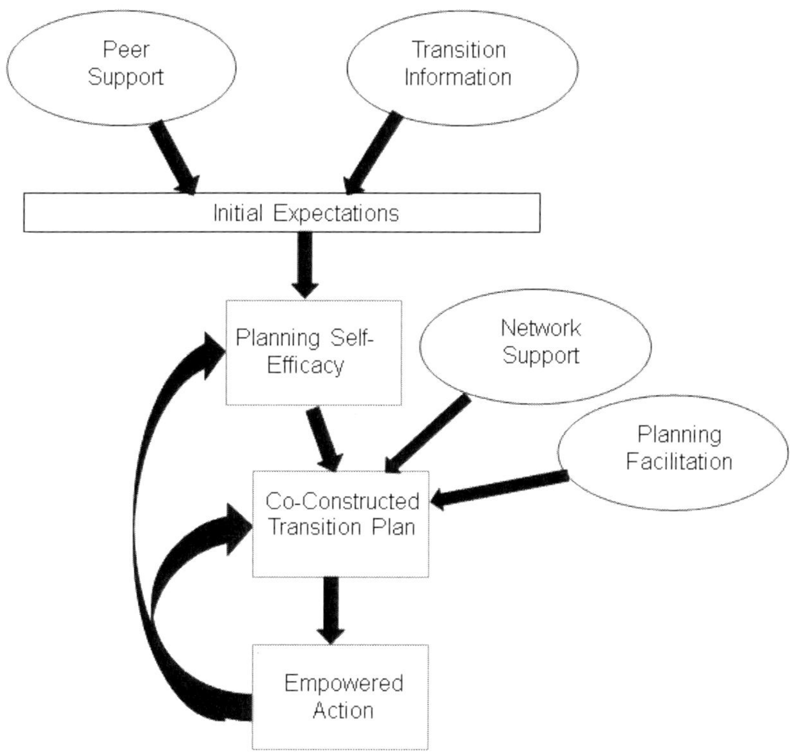

Figure 1. A Theory of Parent Empowerment in Transition Planning.

As depicted in Figure 1, enhanced parent participation in transition planning can be viewed as a two-stage process. The initial experience that laid the groundwork for empowerment was becoming aware of new possibilities for their children's future. For many parents, these new possibilities went well beyond their previous conception of the limited set of services or opportunities that they thought would be available beyond high school. Envisioning new possibilities also included a clearer focus on what their child could do rather than on what he or she could not do, and information about combining formal and informal supports and using formal supports in innovative ways. And during this stage, parent-to-parent peer support is especially valuable in creating a shared awareness that a positive future is achievable.

Background information and peer support creates a platform on which to begin to build a transition plan. This point in the process might be termed "planning self-efficacy," because families felt at this point that they had the confidence and resources to move forward. Initial expectations may also play a role in determining whether or not planning self-efficacy is achieved. The one family whose momentum towards implementing a transition plan ended when the project intervention ended began with an expectation that transition planning was essentially a professional service, and thus their focus centered exclusively on applying for services, waiting for eligibility to be determined, and so on. The project was not powerful enough to offset those expectations.

Once a critical level of planning self-efficacy is attained, a second stage of individualized follow-along assistance identifies and helps manage the multiple tasks involved in making and implementing a transition plan. At this point a skilled facilitator is especially valuable. The facilitator both guides families through this process and also models a spirit of tenacity and perseverance that is needed in working towards transition goals.

Another key component of this second stage of the empowerment process is enlisting the help of informal resources such as friends, relatives, neighbors, community members and organizations. Learning that there are others with new perspectives and access to new resources who could help share responsibility for implementing transition tasks helps make the process manageable. In addition, it helps parents envision a future life when a broader support system surrounds their adult child and they are not the only source of support.

Parents also benefit from seeing their child contributing to the transition plan, and as dealing successfully with a certain amount of anxiety in relation to discussing his or her future, in ways that they may not have appreciated before. Families know from years of experience what works, what disrupts their child and the family's equilibrium, and that if things go wrong, if the process creates too much anxiety, for example, they are going to be the ones left to pick up the pieces. But as parents see that youth with ASD are accomplishing new things and experiencing success, they develop a more strength-based perspective, and youth themselves feel more empowered. These processes seem to reinforce one another and combine to challenge previous conceptions about what was possible. As a result, they allow the co-construction of a transition plan by the parent and student, and lead to active efforts to implement the plan. Meeting over the course of several months, the planning team examines the results of initial exploration or advocacy activities, and this may result in plan revisions.

Conclusion

Students and families welcome the opportunity to be more centrally involved in transition planning, and such involvement leads to more positive post-school outcomes than the traditional professionally-driven processes. The three-component Family-Centered Transition Planning model is an intervention that provides students and families with critical support, including the information and planning facilitation needed to direct the transition process. And the model appears to be flexible enough to allow for a variety of modifications to respond to individual needs.

Summary and Lessons Learned

Data from four-years of Family-Centered Transition Planning implementation showed that FCTP has a positive impact on the future expectations that transitioning students have for themselves and their parents have for them, and on students' level of vocational decision-making and self-determination. Follow-up interviews found that greater percentages of FCTP participants were working and participating in postsecondary education than has been reported for any other intervention. An analysis of student and family expectations showed that one of the most important benefits of FCTP is its role in helping students and their families to be "on the same page" in their views of transition tasks and objectives.

A qualitative study of the perspectives of the parents of students with ASD found that the combination of group training and individualized planning sessions helped break the process into manageable steps and made families aware of a wider array of available resources and supports, and thus changed their perspectives on what was possible for their adult child. And parents were impressed with how actively their children were able to participate when the process was geared to their needs and provisions were made to make planning accessible to them. Particularly noteworthy was the way students with ASD were able to handle a controlled degree of anxiety in relation to transition topics. Allowing youth to experience some of the tension and anxiety that is typical during adolescence in our culture was part of a process of growth and maturity towards a greater level of choice and responsibility.

When implementing transition plans involved making requests of schools and adult service agencies, the responses were mixed. Some schools responded positively and creatively, but other schools were unresponsive; and in one case, failed to even acknowledge the plan that they had developed. Adult service providers were even less supportive, with all families involved with Vocational Rehabilitation agencies viewing the experience negatively. This finding is problematic given the importance of active collaboration among service providers in the transition process. Increased student and family empowerment must be matched by increased flexibility and responsiveness on the part of schools and adult service systems. More research is also needed on strategies for engaging schools and adult service systems to become effective partners with students and families in the transition process.

Sustainability and Future Directions

Significant improvements in student outcomes were maintained when implementation shifted to community service providers with one exception. While both parent expectations and vocational decision-making showed similar levels of improvement before and after community provider involvement in implementation, student expectations improved, but not to a significant degree. It may be that facilitators external to the project were not as skilled in working with individuals on the spectrum to expand their views of the possibilities for adulthood. It may also be that, when referral sources are required to pay for a service, they tend to refer individuals with a history of more negative experiences, with whom the intervention was less effective. And it should be noted that community implementation outcomes remain significantly better than those resulting from the usual transition planning.

Further research is required to examine this issue.

And sustainability efforts for FCTP remain a work in progress. By the end of year four, no community organization had taken full control over implementation, or developed funding sources sufficient to sustain the project. In an environment where service demands far exceed available resources, it may unfortunately be unrealistic to expect that thoughtful advance planning and full involvement of students and families are high priorities. A longer time period may also be needed to achieve substantial systems change. And this will involve addressing at least four related challenges.

1. FCTP involves a fairly significant time commitment on the part of families, and they need to be "sold" on the benefits before making this type of commitment. Those doing recruitment and enrollment must be intimately familiar with how life-changing the process can be, and be able to communicate this effectively to new families.
2. Planning Facilitators, when working primarily with consumers and families in their own homes, can feel disconnected from organizational supports. And their role is sometimes difficult to negotiate (for example, when parents disagree with one another and each tries to get the facilitator to "take sides"). Methods of mentoring, sustaining and supporting facilitators need to be further developed as part of sustainability efforts.
3. Community service provider organizations with a proven track record of service provision and contracts with schools and other funding organizations are the most logical choice as host organizations for FCTP. But such organizations are designed to please their customers – those providing their funds – and thus are wary of getting involved in any activity where they could be in the middle of a conflict or disagreement. Although FCTP does not involve direct advocacy on behalf of families for any specific funds or services, it is easy for an organization providing FCTP to become indirectly unconnected, or to be perceived as connected, to various requests to and disputes with funders. It might therefore be best if FCTP providers do not provide any other services.
4. Asking two or more organizations to jointly fund a service involves a host of logistical problems. Despite a long-standing national focus on interagency transition collaboration, in practice most of these organizations have no mechanism for jointly serving the same person at the same time. It may take many months before someone referred by funder #1 also becomes a client of funder #2. And each organization has its own standard procedures and service offerings. Adding a third organization to the mix complicates matters still further. It may be necessary to accept that a single funding source will pay the full fee for FCTP. And this should also include provisions for families with sufficient resources to self-pay.

Another modification worth investigating is whether school transition coordinators (or those in similar roles, e.g., case manager) can embed FCTP, or aspects of it, into their work. There are several dangers to this approach, including a high probability that the results will be "watered down" from the pure FCTP model, but this may prove to be the most sustainable way to move FCTP up to scale.

Students and families have a strong interest in greater control over the transition to adult life, and increased involvement in planning has the potential to play a central and powerful role in creating positive futures for transitioning students with ASD. Future efforts should focus on developing a variety of options for planning processes that are truly family-centered, as well as continuing efforts to sustain implementation in diverse communities with existing funding resources.

References

Adreon, D., & Durocher, J. S. (2007). Evaluating the college transition needs of individuals with high-functioning autism spectrum disorders. *Intervention in School & Clinic, 42*, 271-279.

Billstedt, E., Gillberg, I. C., & Gillberg, C. (2011). Aspects of quality of life in adults diagnosed with autism in childhood. *Autism, 15*(1), 7-20.

Bourke-Taylor, H., Howie, L. & Law, M. (2012). Impact of caring for a school-aged child with a disability: Understanding mothers' perspectives. *Australian Occupational Therapy Journal, 57,* 127-136.

Briel, L. W., & Getzel, E. E. (2009). Postsecondary options for students with autism. In P. Wehman, M. Smith & C. Schall (Eds.), *Autism and the transition to adulthood: Success beyond the classroom* (pp. 189-207). Baltimore, MD: Paul H. Brookes.

Camarena, P. M., & Sarigiani, P. A. (2009). Postsecondary educational aspirations of high-functioning adolescents with autism spectrum disorders and their parents. *Focus on Autism and Other Developmental Disabilities, 24*, 115-128.

Carrington, S., Templeton, E., & Papinczak, T. (2003). Adolescents with Asperger Syndrome and perceptions of friendship. *Focus on Autism & Other Developmental Disabilities, 18*(4), 211-218.

Carter, E., Trainor, A., Cakiroglu, O., Swedeen, & Owens, L. (2010). Availability of and access to career development activities for transition-age youth with disabilities. *Career Development for Exceptional Individuals*, 33, 13-24.

Cederlund, M., Hagberg, B., Billstedt, E., Gillberg, I., & Gillberg, C. (2008). Asperger Syndrome and autism: A comparative longitudinal follow-up study more than 5 years after original diagnosis. *Journal of Autism & Developmental Disorders, 38*(1), 72-85.

Certo, N., & Luecking, R. (2011). Transition and employment: Reflections from a 40 year perspective. *Journal of Vocational Rehabilitation, 35*, 157-161.

Certo, N., Mautz, D., Pumpian, I., Sax, K., Smalley, H., Wade, D., & Batterman, N. (2003). A review and discussion of a model for seamless transition to adulthood. *Education and Training in Developmental Disabilities 38*(1), 15-20.

Chambers, C. R., Hughes, C., & Carter, E. W. (2004). Parent and sibling perspectives on transition to adulthood. *Education and Training in Developmental Disabilities, 39*(2), 79-94.

Chiang, H.-M., Cheung, Y. K., Li, H., & Tsai, L. Y. (2013). Factors associated with participation in employment for high school leavers with autism. *Journal of Autism and Developmental Disorders, 43*(8), 1832-1842.

Cimera, R., & Burgess, S. (2011). Do adults with autism benefit monetarily from working in their communities? *Journal of Vocational Rehabilitation, 34*, 173-180.

Cimera, R., Burgess, S., & Wiley, A. (2013). Does providing transition services early enable students with ASD to achieve better outcomes as adults? *Research and Practice for Persons with Severe Disabilities, 38*, 88-93.

Clare, L. & Garnier, H. (2000). Parents' goals for adolescents diagnosed with developmental delays in early childhood. *Journal of Early Adolescence, 20*, 442-466.

Cobb, B., & Alwell, M. (2009). Transition planning/coordinating interventions for youth with disabilities: A systematic review. *Career Development for Exceptional Individuals, 32*(2), 70-81.

DeFur, S. (2003). IEP transition planning: From compliance to quality. *Exceptionality, 11*, 115-128.

Deguara, M., Jelasi, O., Micallef, B., & Callus, A. (2012). How we like to live when we have the chance. *British Journal of Learning Disabilities, 40*, 123-127.

Eaves, L., & Ho, H. (2008). Young adult outcome of Autism Spectrum Disorders. *Journal of Autism and Developmental Disorders, 38*(4), 739-747.

Edmondson, C., & Cain, H. (2003). The spirit of the Individuals with Disabilities Education Act: Collaboration between special education and vocational rehabilitation for the transition of students with disabilities. *Journa of Applied Rehabilitation, 33*(4), 10-14.

Fixsen, D., Naoom, S., Blasé, K., Friedman, R. & Wallace, F (2005). *Implementation research: A synthesis of the literature.* Tampa, FL: Univ. of S, Florida Louis de la Parte Mental Health Institute (Publication No. 231).

Germeijs, V., & Verscheren, K. (2009). Adolescents' career decision-making process: Related to quality of attachment to parents? *Journal of Research on Adolescence, 19*, 459-483.

Gray, K., Keating, C., Taffe, J., Brereton, A., Einfeld, S., Reardon, T., & Tonge, B. (2014). Adult outcomes in autism: Community inclusion and living skills. *Journal of Autism and Developmental Disorders*, Retrieved December 28, 2014 from http://dx.doi.org/10.1007/s10803-014-2159-x

Green, S. (2007). "We're tired, not sad": Benefits and burdens of mothering a child with a disability. *Social Science and Medicine, 64*, 150-163.

Hagner, D. & Kurtz, A. (in review). Changes in expectations and vocational decision-making following family-centered transition planning. *Focus on Autism and Other Developmental Disabilities.*

Hagner, D., Kurtz, A., Cloutier, H., Arakelian, C., Brucker, D. & May, J. (2012). Outcomes of a family-centered transition process for students with autism spectrum disorders. *Focus on Autism and Other Developmental Disabilities, 27,* 42-50.

Hagner, D., Kurtz, A., May, J. & Cloutier, H. (2014). Person-centered planning for transition-aged youth with autism spectrum disorders. *Journal of Rehabilitation, 80* (1), 4-10.

Hendricks, D. (2010). Employment and adults with autism spectrum disorders: Challenges and strategies for success. *Journal of Vocational Rehabilitation, 32*(2), 125-134.

Hetherington, S. A., Durant-Jones, L., Johnson, K., Nolan, K., Smith, E., Taylor-Brown, S., & Tuttle, J. (2010). The lived experiences of adolescents with disabilities and their parents in transition planning. *Focus on Autism & Other Developmental Disabilities, 25*(3), 163-172.

Holburn, S., Jacobson, J., Schwartz, A., Flory, , & Vietze, P. (2004). The Willowbrook Futures Project: A Longitudinal analysis of person-centered planning. *American Journal on Mental Retardation, 109*, 63-76.

Holmes, D., & Chaffee, K. (2007). Transition planning for individuals with autism spectrum disorder (ASD). *Rehabilitation of individuals with autism spectrum disorders* (pp. 15-36). Washington, DC.

Holmes, D., & Shore, S. (2005). *Adults with autism.* Bethesda, MD: Interagency Autism Coordinating Council.

Holwerda, A., van der Klink, J. J., Groothoff, J. W., & Brouwer, S. (2012). Predictors for work participation in individuals with an autism spectrum disorder: A systematic review. *Journal of Occupational Rehabilitation, 22*(3), 333-352.

Howlin, P., Goode, S., Hutton, J., & Rutter, M. (2004). Adult outcome for children with autism. *Journal of Child Psychology & Psychiatry, 45*(2), 212-229.

Howlin, P. (2013). Social disadvantage and exclusion: adults with autism lag far behind in employment prospects. *Journal of the American Academy of Child and Adolescent Psychiatry, 52*, 897-899.

Ivey, J. K. (2004). What do parents expect? A study of likelihood and importance issues for children with autism spectrum disorders. *Focus on Autism & Other Developmental Disabilities, 19*(1), 27-33.

Kim, K., & Yurnbull, A. (2004). Transition to adulthood for students with severe intellectual disabilities: Shifting toward person--family interdependent planning. *Research and Practice for Persons with Severe Disabilities, 29*, 53-57.

Kraemer, B., & Blacher, J. (2001). Transition for young adults with severe mental retardation: School preparation, parent expectations, and family involvement. *Mental Retardation, 39*, 423-435.

Landmark, L. J., Song, J., & Dalun, Z. (2010). Substantiated best practices in transition: Fifteen plus years later. *Career Development for Exceptional Individuals, 33*(3), 165-176.

Lecavalier, L., Snow, A., & Norris, M. (2011). Autism spectrum disorders and intellectual disability. *International handbook of autism and pervasive developmental disorders* (pp. 37-51). New York NY: Springer.

Liptak, G. S., Kennedy, J. A., & Dosa, N. P. (2011). Social participation in a nationally representative sample of older youth and young adults with autism. *Journal of Developmental and Behavioral Pediatrics, 32*(4), 277-283.

Locke, J., Ishijima, E. H., Kasari, C., & London, N. (2010). Loneliness, friendship quality and the social networks of adolescents with high-functioning autism in an inclusive school setting. *Journal of Research in Special Educational Needs, 10*(2), 74-81.

McGovern, C. W., & Sigman, M. (2005). Continuity and change from early childhood to adolescence in autism. *Journal of Child Psychology & Psychiatry, 46*(4), 401-408.

Migliore, A., & Lugas, J. (2011). Students with autism: Setting higher expectations for postsecondary education *DataNote Series (Vol. 48)*. Boston, MA: Institute for Community Inclusion.

Migliore, A., & Zalewska, A. (2012). What are the employment experiences of youth with autism after high school? (Vol. 49). Boston, MA: Institute for Community Inclusion.

Newman, L., Wagner, M., Knokey, A.-M., Marder, C., Nagle, K., Shaver, D., et al. (2011). *The Post-High School Outcomes of Young Adults With Disabilities up to 8 Years After High School. A Report From the National Longitudinal Transition Study-2 (NLTS2)* (NCSER 2011-3005). Menlo Park, CA: SRI International.

Powers, K., Geenen, S., & Powers, L. (2009). Similarities and differences in the transition expectations of youth and parents. *Career Development for Exceptional Individuals, 32*, 132-144.

Revell, G., & Miller, L. A. (2009). Navigating the world of adult services and benefits planning. In P. Wehman, M. D. Smith & C. Schall (Eds.), *Autism and the transition to adulthood: Success beyond the classroom* (pp. 139-162). Baltimore, MD: Paul H. Brookes.

Roberts, K. D. (2010). Topic areas to consider when planning transition from high school to postsecondary education for students with autism spectrum disorders. *Focus on Autism and Other Developmental Disabilities, 25*, 158-162.

Robertson, J., Emerson, E., Hatton, C., Elliott, J., McIntosh, B., Swift, P., & Joyce, T. (2006). Longitudinal analysis of the impact and cost of person-centered planning for people with intellectual disabilities in England. *American Journal on Mental Retardation, 111*, 400-416.

Roest, A., Dubas, J., & Gerris, J. (2009). Value transmissions between fathers, mothers, and adolescent and emerging adult children: The role of family climate. *Journal of Family Psychology, 23*, 146-155.

Roux, A. M., Shattuck, P., Cooper, B. P., Anderson, K. A., Wagner, M., & Narendorf, S. C. (2013). Postsecondary employment experiences among young adults with an autism spectrum disorder. *Journal of the American Academy of Child and Adolescent Psychiatry, 52*(9), 931-939.

Russa, M. B., Matthews, A. L., & Owen-DeSchryver, J. S. (2014). Expanding supports to Improve the lives of families of children with Autism Spectrum Disorder. *Journal of Positive Behavior Interventions*, Retrieved December 28, 2014 from http://pbi.sagepub.com/content/early/2014/04/28/1098300714532134.full.pdf+html

Ruppar, A. L., & Gaffney, J. S. (2011). Individualized Education Program team decisions: A preliminary study of conversations, negotiations, and power. *Research and Practice for Persons with Severe Disabilities, 36*(1-2), 11-22.

Schall, C. (2009). Educational and transition planning. In P. Wehman, M. D. Smith & C. Schall (Eds.), *Autism and the transition to adulthood: Success beyond the classroom* (pp. 39-93). Baltimore, MD: Paul H. Brookes.

Shattuck, P., Wagner, M., Narendorf, S., Sterzing, P., & Hensley, M. (2011). Post-high school service use among young adults with an autism spectrum disorder. *Archives of Pediatrics and Adolescent Medicine, 165*(2), 141.

Shattuck, P., Narendorf, S. C., Cooper, B., Sterzing, P. R., Wagner, M., & Taylor, J. L. (2012). (2012). Postsecondary education and employment among youth with autism spectrum disorder. *Journal of Pediatrics*, *129*, 6, 1042-1049.

Shogren, K. A., & Plotner, A. J. (2012). Transition planning for students with intellectual disability, autism, or other disabilities: Data from the National Longitudinal Transition Study-2. *Intellectual and developmental disabilities, 50*(1), 16-30.

Shogren, K. A., Wehmeyer, M., Palmer, S. B., Soukup, J., Garner, N., & Lawrence, M. (2007). Examining individual and ecological predictors of the self-determination of students with disabilities. *Exceptional Children, 73*(4), 488-509.

Targett, P. S., & Smith, M. D. (2009). Living in the community. In P. Wehman, M. D. Smith & C. Schall (Eds.), *Understanding the transition from school to adulthood for students with autism* (pp. 233-250). Baltimore, MD: Paul H. Brookes.

Targett, P. S., & Wehman, P. (2009). Integrated employment. In P. Wehman, M. D. Smith & C. Schall (Eds.), *Understanding the transition from school to adulthood for students with autism* (pp. 163-188). Baltimore, MD: Paul H. Brookes.

Taylor, J. L., & Mailick, M. R. (2014). A longitudinal examination of 10-year change in vocational and educational activities for adults with autism spectrum disorders. *Developmental Psychology, 50*(3), 699-708.

Taylor, J., & Seltzer, M. (2010). Employment and post-secondary educational activities for young adults with autism spectrum disorders during the transition to adulthood. *Journal of Autism and Developmental Disorders, 41*, 566-574.

Taylor, J., Smith, L., & Mailick, M. (2014). Engagement in vocational activities promotes behavioral development for adults with Autism Spectrum Disorders. *Journal of Autism and Developmental Disorders, 44*, 1447-1460.

Tehee, E., Honan, R. & Hevey, D. (2009). Factors contributing to stress in parents of individuals with Autistic Spectrum Disorders. *Journal of Applied Research in Intellectual Disabilities, 22*, 34-42.

Test, D. W., Mazzotti, V. L., Mustian, A. L., Fowler, C. H., Kortering, L., & Kohler, P. (2009). Evidence-based secondary transition predictors for improving postschool outcomes for students with disabilities. *Career Development for Exceptional Individuals, 32*(3), 160-181.

Test, D. W., Smith, L. E., & Carter, E. W. (2014). Equipping youth with autism spectrum disorders for adulthood: Promoting rigor, relevance, and relationships. *Remedial and Special Education, 35*(2), 80-90.

Tiffany, R. (2004). Review of the Vocational Decision-Making Interview – Revised. *14th mental measurements yearbook.*

VanBergeijk, E., Klin, A., & Volkmar, F. (2008). Supporting more able students on the autism spectrum: College and beyond. *Journal of Autism & Developmental Disorders, 38*, 1359-1370.

Wagner, M., Newman, L., Cameto, P., Levine, P., & Garza, N. (2006). *An overview of findings from wave 2 of the National Longitudinal Transition Study-2.* Washington DC: National Center for Special Education Research.

Waisman Center. (2009). *Medical home service system guidelines for autism spectrum disorders.* Retrieved May 10. 2009, from http://www.waisman.wisc.edu/nmhai/

Wehmeyer, M., & Kelchner, K. (1995). *The Arc's Self-Determination Scale.* Arlington, TX: Arc National Headquarters.

Wei, X., Wagner, M., Hudson, L., Jennifer, W. Y., & Shattuck, P. (2014). Transition to adulthood employment, education, and disengagement in individuals with Autism Spectrum Disorders. *Emerging Adulthood,*

Retrieved December 29, 2014 from http://eax.sagepub.com/content/early/2014/05/13/2167696814534417.full.pdf+html.

Wittenburg, D. C., Golden, T., & Fishman, M. (2002). Transition options for youth with disabilities: An overview of the programs and policies that affect the transition from school. *Journal of Vocational Rehabilitation, 17*(3), 195-206.

Wolman, J., Campeau, P., DuBois, P., Mithaug, D. & Stolarski, V. (1994). *AIR Self-determination scale and user guide*. New York: Teachers' College Press.

Wong, M. & Heriot, S. (2007). Vicarious futurity in autism and childhood dementia. *Journal of Autism and Developmental Disorders, 37*, 1833-1841.

Young, R., Marshall, S., Dornene, J., Graham, M., Logan, C., Zaidman, A., et al. (2008). Transition to adulthood as a parent-youth project: Governance transfer, career promotion, and relational processes. *Journal of Counseling Psychology, 55*, 297-307.

In: Autism Spectrum Disorders
Editor: Arlene Valdez
ISBN: 978-1-63482-547-4

Chapter 4

Social Experiences of Male Adults with Autism Spectrum Disorders

Efrosini Kalyva[1] and Vlastaris Tsakiris[2]
[1]Senior Lecturer, The International Faculty of the University of Sheffield, City College, Thessaloniki, Greece
[2]"Learning through play", Diagnostic and Rehabilitation Centre, Thessaloniki, Greece

Abstract

Most research in the area of autism spectrum disorders has concentrated on children and adolescents, while very few studies have been conducted on adults with autism spectrum disorders (especially those diagnosed in adulthood). The aim of this qualitative study is to explore the experiences of adults with autism spectrum disorders with a focus on their social relationships. Six of the men who participated in the study were diagnosed with autism spectrum disorders in late childhood or in their teens, while the remaining four received a diagnosis in their adulthood (up to 4 years prior to the study). The diagnoses of autism spectrum disorders were made by public local educational authorities or hospital clinics by multidisciplinary teams comprising of psychiatrists, psychologists, speech therapists, occupational therapists, and social workers. Two of them lived on their own, five were living with their parents and/or siblings and the remaining three had their own families. They were interviewed by the researchers for 1.5 hours using an in-depth semi-structured format and content analysis was used to analyse and interpret their thoughts and experiences. The themes that emerged from the analysis are: coming to terms with the diagnosis; revealing the diagnosis to their family/spouse, friends and colleagues; initiating and maintaining social relationships (challenges and facilitators); the impact of culture. This is among the first qualitative studies looking at the social experiences of adults with autism spectrum disorders. Therefore, it has certain limitations such as its constrained generalization to female adults with autism spectrum disorders or males from different cultures.

Introduction

Poor social functioning constitutes a core deficit of autism spectrum disorders. According to the DSM-V (American Psychiatric Association, 2013), the social deficit in autism spectrum disorders is marked by impairment in the use of nonverbal behaviors, failure to develop peer relationships, a lack of seeking to share enjoyment, interests, or achievements with others, and a general lack of social or emotional reciprocity.

Baron Cohen and Wheelright (2003) compared adolescents and adults with high-functioning autism spectrum disorders with typically developing peers and found that the former engage in less close, less empathic, less supportive, and less meaningful social relationships.

Most adults with autism spectrum disorders experience difficulties with their social skills (Seltzer, Krauss, Shattuck, Orsmond, Swe, and Lord, 2003). Howlin, Mawhood, and Rutter (2000) followed-up a group of 19 individuals with autism spectrum disorders into their adulthood and found that only three (16%) had one or more friends of roughly their own age with whom they shared various interests and social activities. Almost half of them (47%) did not have any particular friends to share activities with. Orsmond, Krauss and Seltzer (2004) reached similar conclusions, with 50% of their sample reporting no peer relationships outside of pre-arranged settings (such as school, work, or other arranged social groups). Moreover, in the same year (2004) Howlin and her group published yet another study with similar findings that corroborate the 2000 study.

Orsmond et al. (2004) found that adults with autism spectrum disorders engage less often in casual social activities (e.g.,, socializing with relatives, friends, neighbors, or school and work friends). When they do decide to engage in such activities they are often facilitated by family members, teachers or service providers. They also point out the lack of information on the level and type of individual motivation that is needed to participate in casual social activities and this is one of the objectives of the present study. Moreover, Orsmond et al. (2004) highlighted the necessity of conducting studies to obtain information directly from individuals with autism spectrum disorders about their own perspectives of their social lives, which is what the present study has attempted to do. It is the first qualitative study to our knowledge to explore the social experiences of male adults with autism spectrum disorders.

Design Overview

In an effort to unveil the social relationship experiences of male adults with autism spectrum disorders, in-depth interviews were conducted with ten participants (Padgett, 1998). The interviews centered around two primary questions: (1) How are their social relationships and skills affected by their autism spectrum disorders? and (2) Which are the factors that facilitate or impede their social relationships? Numerous probes requesting examples, clarification or further information about topics such as friendships, colleagues, intimate romantic relationships etc. were used throughout the interviews.

Recruitement Procedures

Interview participants were recruited from a therapeutic and rehabilitation center for children and adolescents with developmental disabilities, which is located in Thessaloniki (Greece) and provides monthly services to more than 100 children and their families. Eight young males who were receiving counseling services at the center were approached and debriefed about the project. Six of them expressed an interest to participate in the study and were given more information together with the informed consents that they had to sign and return to the researchers in order to participate. Despite the fact that they were adults (aged 18-23 years old) and they had normal IQs, because of their diagnosed disability oral ascent was solicited also from their parents. The remaining four males with autism spectrum disorders who took part in this study were fathers of children and adolescents with autism spectrum disorders who were receiving treatment at the centre. They were diagnosed in adulthood after their child was diagnosed because they could identify similar symptoms in themselves.

A minimum time of four years since diagnosis was a prerequisite for inclusion in the study. Out of the 7 fathers who have disclosed their disability to the researchers and were informed about this study, 4 agreed to participate and signed informed consent forms. All the participants have received their diagnosis of autism spectrum disorders from public clinical or educational settings from multidisciplinary teams using different assessments. For the purpose of this study their diagnosis of autism spectrum disorders was confirmed using ADOS-G2 and the revised DSM-V criteria. Approval for this research was obtained from the Center's Ethics Committee. There was no monetary compensation for participation in the research, but all the information would be used to identify some themes that would be discussed during six complimentary individual and/or family therapy sessions.

Data Collection

Interviews with the participants were scheduled to take place either while their children were in therapy or when their own therapy was scheduled, since this was agreed to be the most convenient option for all parties involved. In the case of the latter, they were not charged for the particular counseling session. All participants had up to two hours at their disposal for the semi-structured face-to face interview. They were informed that they could refrain from answering at any time or discontinue the interview and still be entitled to the free counseling sessions. However, no such issues occurred. Examples of interview questions include: "How do you interact with your friends on a social basis?" "How do you inform others about your disability?" "What helps you interact better with others?" and "What is the most difficult part of interacting with others?". Both researchers are trained to work with individuals with autism spectrum disorders and their families on social issues for more than a decade. At the end of the interviews the researchers went through some key points with them and asked them if their opinions were accurately recorded and interpreted. All participants were assured of their confidentiality.

All the interviews were recorded and notes were kept with the participants' permission. Audio records were kept safe in a personal computer in an office under an assumed file and were erased after the transcription. The average approximate duration of the interviews was 1 hour and 15 min (ranging from 53 min to 1 h and 32 min).

Content analysis was used to identify the themes from the interview transcripts (Patton, 2002). Two coders analyzed and coded the transcripts using a frequency count strategy to calculate the number of times a participant mentioned each identified theme. This technique serves as a guard against both respondent and investigator bias (Miles and Huberman, 1994) and as an indication of interrater reliability (which was as high as 92.5%) for this study. The few remaining differences were resolved through discussion among the coders.

Results

The age of the participants ranged from 18 to 46 years old, with males diagnosed in adulthood being older than males diagnosed in childhood or adolescence. Two of the participants were living on their own (one was divorced with a child with autism spectrum disorders), five were living with their parents and/or siblings and the remaining three had their own families. Two fathers were employed and the other two were unemployed. Out of the six younger participants four were studying and the remaining two were looking for a job. Employing the analytic strategy described above, four content-related themes about social experiences were identified. They include: coming to terms with the diagnosis; revealing the diagnosis to family/spouse, friends and colleagues; initiation and maintenance of social relationships (challenges and facilitators); as well as the impact of culture.

Content-Related Themes

Coming to Terms with the Diagnosis

A primary theme that emerged from the interviews was that male adults with autism spectrum disorders have difficulties coming to terms with the diagnosis regardless of when it was made (childhood, adolescence or adulthood). All the participants agreed that it was a relief to get a diagnosis, since it helped them make sense of what was happening to them. An 18-year-old man reported that ‘I found out that I had autism spectrum disorders when I was 13. I was misdiagnosed with ADHD. I even received mediation for that. I knew I was different from the others. Then I understood why. Not immediately, of course. They told me what autism spectrum disorders were. Then it made sense'. A 39 year-old man said 'I had to know the truth. Am I like my son? We have so many things in common as characters. He does not communicate well, though. And he is 6 years old'.

All the participants agreed that getting a diagnosis was a difficult and even humiliating experience that they would rather leave behind. A 20-year-old man said 'They thought I was stupid. They kept measuring this and that trying to understand why I behave this way. They never bothered to ask me. My parents took me everywhere. Tests and more tests… the worst being talking about me as if I were not present'. A 42-year-old man revealed that 'I sort of felt I had to go. My wife was putting a lot of pressure on me. We had to wait for months to get an appointment, we paid a lot of money, and most 'experts' were not even trained to diagnose autism spectrum disorders. They were just reading and ticking lists'.

It took most of them a substantial amount of time to come to terms with the diagnosis, even though it did help them understand why they behave or feel in a certain way. One of the main reasons was that they had a different conceptualization of what autism spectrum disorders means. A 21 year-old man said that he did not want to believe that he has autism spectrum disorders because 'one child with autism spectrum disorders I knew was screaming all the time and moving his arms. He was not able to talk and he went to a special school and he was also slow. When I heard I had autism spectrum disorders too, I thought no way. I am not like him… it took me months to accept it and many fights with my parents'. A 46-year-old man was not convinced of the diagnosis because he did not meet the criteria. In his own words 'I searched the Internet and I found many lists of symptoms. A lot of them do not apply to me. I have a family. I am smart. I have a good job and I make a lot of money. I could not do all that if I had autism spectrum disorders. I thought they were wrong. But then I talked to you and you explained about the spectrum and what it means. I could identify with the examples that you gave me. However, I still believe it is a nightmare that we will get out of'.

Despite the fact that all the participants stated that they had by now come to terms with their diagnosis of autism spectrum disorders, most of them experienced difficulties sharing it with others (even close family members and friends). This leads to the second theme that derived from the analysis.

Revealing the Diagnosis to Family/Spouse or Friends

All the participants agreed that they did not have to reveal the diagnosis to their family/spouse, since they were involved in the diagnostic process from the beginning. In the case of the young males who were diagnosed in their childhood or teen years, their parents initiated the diagnostic process. Actually, their parents were told of the diagnosis even before they were and this meant in practice that the parents revealed the diagnosis to their children and not the other way around. Older men were also encouraged by their spouses to consult an expert and get a diagnosis (even in the case of the divorced father), because they felt that it would help them get closure. One wife told her 46-year-old husband that 'she needs to find out why I behave this way. Why I can be so understanding and so cruel at the same time. Why I can see only black and white. And even more important how to work on it'.

Sharing the news with the wider family was another issue. Two of the participants stated that their parents informed the wider family about their children's disability once they got the diagnosis. A 19-year-old remembers that 'during a family celebration my parents told the rest that I was diagnosed with autism spectrum disorders, without even asking me. They said it out loud, described what it means and then asked if anybody had questions. Nobody asked anything. They were just looking at me. Nobody ever mentioned it again!'. The rest of the participants consulted with their parents/spouses and decided to share the new with others gradually and to avoid announcing it, unless any questions were raised. A 23-year-old remembers his mother saying that 'nobody can tell that I have autism spectrum disorders. So, why tell them? Only if they ask a lot and insist. There is no point looking for trouble. And my father nodded'.

Similar trends were recorded when it came to revealing the diagnosis to friends and or/colleagues. The two participants who revealed their disability to their family were encouraged by their parents to talk openly to their friends. A 19-year-old remembers his anguish because 'I did not know exactly what to tell them. I had discussed it with my parents, but they were not there to help me. What if they asked me something that I did not know? ... I was just learning about autism spectrum disorders myself... It was OK. They were cool... They hugged me'. The rest of the participants followed the same tactic and told others only if needed. A 42-year-old man had to tell his boss because 'I had problems socializing with colleagues. I did not want him to think I was a snob'. A 23-year-old revealed the diagnosis to a friend because 'I knew I was going to lose him. He got tired of me talking about my own interests, putting myself first, forgetting to call to see how he is... Now he knows it's better. It's our secret. Best friends share secrets'.

Then, we asked the 4 fathers who were diagnosed in adulthood to explain why they shared their diagnosis with us, when they had decided against telling other people. They told us that it was because we were working with their children with autism spectrum disorders and they knew that we could tell. Therefore, there was no point lying. One father said that he felt it would help to give him advice on how to deal with his personal issues, although he did not believe that he needed counseling himself. Another father said that he had come to trust us over the years that we were working with his son with autism spectrum disorders and he knew we would understand. The documented difficulty to reveal the diagnosis to family, friends, and colleagues is one of the greatest obstacles in initiating and maintaining social relationships, as is the focus of the third theme.

Initiation and Maintenance of Social Relationships (Challenges and Facilitators)

The participants differentiated between the initiation and the maintenance of social relationships in terms of the challenges and facilitators that they encountered. Most participants agreed that initiating a social contact is less demanding than maintaining it. The six younger males were attending counseling sessions targeting their social skills deficits and they had learned techniques on how to initiate social contact. A 21-year-old said 'I have learned some tricks to approach other people and start a conversation. They work most of the times. But it is hard work. I need to think what to do and what to say all the time. Especially if it is a girl I like…' The older participants have figured out ways of initiating social contact over time mainly through trial and error. As a 35-year-old admits 'I have learned some tricks on the way. I have some opening lines that I have rehearsed and they work. This is how I met my wife'.

All the participants agreed that they should not talk about their disability when initiating a social contact. The parameters that influence the experience of initiating a social contact are:

a. the setting: Being in a noisy and or/unfamiliar place may place an extra burden on the individual with autism spectrum disorders, while a relaxed, quiet and friendly atmosphere can facilitate social initiation. A 19-year-old explained the difficulty of trying to initiate a social contact in a cafeteria 'I try to forget about the noise and remember all the things that I have learned… Very hard… Cannot even hear my own thoughts'. An 18-year-old reported a more positive experience outside the classroom when 'all the others have gone to the restaurant. The other guy was sitting next to me on the bench near the classroom. I asked him something about the class… it worked'.

b. the topic: Most of the participants said that they are reverting to topics that are familiar to them or popular in order to initiate contact, because this makes them feel safer. A 46-year-old said that 'football is a good conversation opener with another guy. It cannot go wrong'. Unfortunately, if it does not work, they may lose their nerve and fail to use a complimentary strategy. As a 35-year-old recalls 'We started talking about PAOK (a football team), but he was not that into sports… I could not think of another topic, so I gradually left his company'.
c. motivation/interest: almost half of the participants mentioned that they usually lack the motivation to initiate a social contact, but they do it because they know they have to. A 23-year-old describes being at a gathering 'where I didn't really want to go, but all the class went. My parents tell me I need to go too and mix with others. It is very time consuming and useless. I know that when I go home, they will start asking me questions…' Most participants also admitted to feel reluctant to initiate a social contact with someone from the opposite sex that they find appealing, because they are afraid of rejection. A 20-year-old described his feelings when seeing a pretty girl at college 'I like … a lot. I try to sit next to her in class. She smiles at me, but doesn't say anything. I know I am supposed to start the conversation. I am the guy. But what if she doesn't like me and starts laughing?'

When probing the participants to talk more about their emotions preceding the initiation of social contact, most said that they feel very anxious and stressed regardless of their age and training. Some of them admitted to practicing the scenario in their heads and trying to act it out as rehearsed, so that nothing goes wrong. Previous negative experiences have troubled most participants and have made them less reluctant to try meeting new people. For some, though, initiating a social contact successfully may be more overwhelming than failing to do so, because of the difficulties of maintaining it. As a 21-year-old puts it 'Once I meet a new person, I get even more stressed. What should I do to keep his interest? What if he thinks I am silly?'

The most difficult social relationships to maintain are with friends and romantic partners for younger participants and with spouses and work colleagues for older participants. The close relationships with parents and siblings are taken for granted for all participants, who do not believe that they need to invest a lot of time and effort in them. The greatest challenges of maintaining social relationships are to control impulses to behave in certain ways; to correctly understand and respond to others' feelings and intentions; to share interests and hobbies; to remain motivated to sustain the relationship; and to overcome disputes and quarrels. Younger participants may be less willing to put some effort in dealing with challenges. An 18-year-old said 'Well, I will try, but they have to try as well. If they do not like me, I will find other friends. Why be pressured?' Older participants are more aware of the sacrifices that they need to make in order to maintain some important relationships in their lives. In the words of a 35-year-old 'I love her (his wife) a lot. It is very hard to understand her at times. And for her to understand me. But, I will not give up… I will keep on trying'.

Some things that can help most of the participants foster social relationships are the social setting and the other person's character. Meeting people in the same place or at regular times (such as work or university) can create a routine that is reassuring for the individual with autism spectrum disorders. A 23-year-old says 'I know that I will see him at the college. We will talk about classes, how we spent the day, what to do later. This makes me feel good'. The other person's accepting personality and positive predisposition can also be crucial to maintaining social relationships as explained by a 40-year-old 'He is always smiling and willing to understand and give me a break. When I get carried away, he will put his hands up in the air, say he gives up and smile. This is enough to bring me back to my senses'.

One of biggest challenges related to maintaining a social contact is whether or not to reveal the diagnosis. Sharing the diagnosis serves a dual purpose. For some individuals, it is an explanation for odd behaviors and according to a 46-year-old 'If I tell others I have autism spectrum disorders, then they will be able to understand why my behavior is a little strange at times'. For some others, it helps them get away with some behaviors. A 19-year-old said that 'When I lose it, I can blame it on autism spectrum disorders. And then others feel bad making a big deal of it'. Most participants agree that sharing the diagnosis is difficult and they refrain from doing it for quite some time, while a few never tell. However, they all agree that disclosing autism spectrum disorders can have a liberating effect. The decision of revealing the diagnosis is largely influenced by culture, as can be seen in the next section.

The Impact of Culture

All the participants argued that living in Greece has an impact on how others perceive and respond to their disability, which in turn influences their social experiences. They believe that the lack of education surrounding disabilities, equal rights and access to education and work are main obstacles for their social lives. A 23-year-old remembers that 'some classmates used to tell me to stop using my disability as an excuse to get marks. They were calling me 'teacher's pet' and they said that if autism spectrum disorders existed, they would have heard about it'. Most participants also admitted that their parents/spouses were ashamed to talk about their disability to family, friends, acquaintances, because in Greece there is stigma associated with disability (especially mental disability). A 40-year-olds says 'My wife asked me not to tell her family. She said they would not understand. It's not like it shows. And they will also ask if I had how come I did not know about it all this time. They have problems accepting that our son has autism spectrum disorders'.

Finally, a widespread belief in Greece is that faith can cure all disorders and diseases and some of the participants were encouraged to go or taken by force to a priest to talk about their autism spectrum disorders. This was thought to be a way to overcome their difficulties, to become more sociable and to acquire friends and wives. A 35-year-old remembers a priest who advised him to marry a religious woman, because she will be able to put up with him.

Conclusion

This was the first qualitative study attempting to explore the social experiences of adult males with autism spectrum disorders. Their social experiences seemed to be affected to a great extent by first coming to terms with the diagnosis and then revealing it to family, friends, and colleagues. Most of the participants agreed that although getting the diagnosis helped them understand why they behave in certain ways, they were disappointed by the long time that it took them to receive the diagnosis and by the whole diagnostic procedure, as found in another study by Kalyva (2012). Similar delays in receiving a diagnosis were recorded by Howlin and Moore in a study that they published in 1997 with parents of 1200 individuals with autism spectrum disorders in the UK. This delay makes some individuals reluctant to accept the diagnosis, since it is often perceived as inadequacy on the part of the mental health professionals involved in the diagnostic process. It is also likely that while individuals with autism spectrum disorders wait to diagnosed, they are reluctant to engage in social interactions because they feel uncertain.

Moreover, since the participants in the present study were at the high-functioning end of the spectrum, they did not present some of the symptoms that are characteristic of autism spectrum disorders. This made them reluctant to accept the diagnosis and is characteristic of the misconceptions that are prevalent in Greece and are caused by the lack of education and the stigmatization associated with autism spectrum disorders (Papageorgiou and Kalyva, 2012). It is worth mentioning that although all the male adults who participated in the study claimed to have accepted their diagnosis, most of them experienced difficulties sharing it with others (even close family members and friends). Since talking about the diagnosis is an essential component of acceptance (Kalyva, 2013), this hesitation to reveal the diagnosis may mean that they have not fully accepted it.

The people who knew about the diagnosis of autism spectrum disorders even before the participants themselves were their parents or their spouses, who were also the ones to encourage them to seek a diagnosis. However, the parents of only two out of the ten male adults with autism spectrum disorders shared the news of their children's diagnosis with family and friends. This was done in a quite unorthodox way and without the consent of the then adolescent with autism spectrum disorders and this is something that should be further researched. When individuals with autism spectrum disorders are able to communicate their thoughts and feelings, they should be actively involved in decision-making regarding when and how the diagnosis will be shared. Family can influence the social life of an adult with autism spectrum disorders, with mothers playing an instrumental role in orchestrating their children's social lives (Orsmond et al., 2004). Therefore, when parents are open about their children's diagnosis, they are more likely to help them plan and expand their social experiences.

All the others parents and spouses advised their children to not talk about their diagnosis, unless they had to. This reflects the lack of education and the fear of stigmatization mentioned above and is characteristic of the stress that family members and individuals with autism spectrum disorders experience when trying to conceal the diagnosis (Kalyva, 2012). Adult males with autism spectrum disorders talked about their disability when they were afraid of losing a friend who could not understand why they behaved oddly, when they needed to justify their behavior to their boss or colleague, and when they thought that the other person already knew about or suspected their disability. The latter was the reason why the older adult participants revealed the diagnosis to the researchers. This fear of sharing the diagnosis with others has a detrimental effect on family life, with parents avoiding taking their children out – especially if they engage in behaviors characteristic of autism spectrum disorders (Papageorgiou and Kalyva, 2010). It is obvious that when individuals with autism spectrum disorders are kept away from family, friends, and peers, they have limited to non-existing opportunities to socialize.

Even though the male participants in this study were not physically isolated from the world, the fear of the revelation of their diagnosis was an important barrier to their social experiences and interactions. When asked to identify which were the factors that obstructed or facilitated their social experiences, they made a distinction between initiating and maintaining a social contact. This distinction is evident also when looking at interventions targeting social skills, where efforts to maintain social interactions are compromised by inadequate skills to initiate social interaction and successful initiations of social interactions are discontinued due to inability to maintain social interactions (Kalyva and Avramidis, 2005).

When it came to initiate social contacts, the younger participants were quite confident, since they were all attending counseling sessions targeting their social skills deficits and they had learned techniques on how to initiate social contact. They mentioned, of course, that it was not always easy to practice what they had learnt, but they had acquired some skills. The older participants who were not receiving any treatment for their autism spectrum disorders have figured out ways of initiating social contact over time mainly through trial and error.

All the participants agreed that they should not talk about their disability when initiating a social contact. On the one hand it makes sense that they do not want to reveal personal information to strangers, but on the other hand this view partly reflects the fear of stigmatization. The parameters that influence the experience of initiating a social contact are the setting, the context and the levels of interest and/or motivation. As far as the setting is concerned, participants argued that being in a noisy and or/unfamiliar place may place an extra burden on the individual with autism spectrum disorders, while a relaxed, quiet and friendly atmosphere can facilitate social initiation. In relation to the topic, most participants said that they had a specific range of topics that they were familiar with or that were considered popular and they used them to initiate social contact. This boosted their self-confidence and their sense of safety, but usually if something went wrong they gave up trying. Finally, as far as interest and or motivation levels are concerned, almost half of the participants mentioned that they usually lack the motivation to initiate a social contact, but they do it because they know they have to. This is consistent with the finding of Orsmond et al. (2004) that individuals with autism spectrum disorders are usually facilitated in their social interactions by family members who emphasize the importance of this interaction. Most participants also admitted to feel reluctant to initiate a social contact with someone from the opposite sex that they find appealing, because they are afraid of rejection. This fear of rejection in combination with limited understanding of social cues can lead to stalking behaviors in adults with autism spectrum disorders and warrant further investigation (Stokes, Newton, and Kaur, 2007).

When probing the participants to talk more about their emotions preceding the initiation of social contact, most said that they feel very anxious and stressed regardless of their age and training. Some of them admitted to practicing the scenario in their heads and trying to act it out as rehearsed, so that nothing goes wrong. Previous negative experiences have troubled most participants and have made them less reluctant to try meeting new people. For some, though, initiating a social contact successfully may be more overwhelming than failing to do so, because of the difficulties of maintaining it. The most difficult social relationships to maintain are with friends and romantic partners for younger participants and with spouses and work colleagues for older participants. The close relationships with parents and siblings are taken for granted for all participants, who do not believe that they need to invest a lot of time and effort in them. The greatest challenges of maintaining social relationships are to control impulses to behave in certain ways; to correctly understand and respond to others' feelings and intentions; to share interests and hobbies; to remain motivated to sustain the relationship; and to overcome disputes and quarrels. Younger participants may be less willing to put some effort in dealing with challenges.

This is the first study that explores the motives and the challenges for engaging in social contacts and interactions, addressing a need that has been identified by Orsmond et al. (2004). All this information should be taken into consideration when planning interventions to address the social skills of individuals with autism spectrum disorders in order to make them more effective. The most popular and effective interventions targeting social skills that could benefit from this information are social stories, the 'circle of friends' and cognitive-behavioral training (Kalyva, 2011; Kalyva, 2012).

This qualitative study, which is the first to explore the social experiences of males with male adults with autism spectrum has certain limitations. To begin with, all the male adults who took part were at the high functioning end of the autism spectrum disorders. Adults with lower levels of functioning might report different experiences, since the level of functional independence and social impairment is linked to participation in social and recreational activities (Orsmond et al., 2004). The findings refer to male adults and they cannot be generalized to females without further investigation, since there is evidence that males and females with autism spectrum disorders think and behave in different ways (Baron-Cohen, 2004). Moreover, this study has taken place in Greece, where certain cultural aspects and practices might have affected the social experiences reported by adult males. The most important cultural influences are stigmatization and lack of education. Therefore, social experiences in different cultures might yield different findings.

Finally, another parameter that should be taken into consideration while interpreting the findings of the present study is that the younger males who participated were attending regular counseling services to improve their social skills among others. There is evidence to suggest that attending psychological services and being educated in inclusive settings enhances participation in social and recreational activities (Orsmond et al., 2004). Therefore, it is likely that less educated males or males who did not receive any treatment could have different social experiences.

This first qualitative study about the social experiences of males with autism spectrum disorders shows that they want to engage in social interactions with others and that they are able to identify and to verbalize the factors that obstruct or facilitate this process. All this preliminary information should be pursued further and incorporated into social skills intervention programs that should target both initiation and maintenance skills to be successful and effective.

References

American Psychiatric Association. (2013). *Diagnostic and statistical manual of mental disorders* (DSM-V) (5th ed.). Washington, DC: American Psychiatric Press.

Baron-Cohen, S. (2004). *Essential difference: Male and female brains and the truth about autism*. Cambridge: Basic Books.

Baron-Cohen, S. and Wheelwright, S. (2003). The Friendship Questionnaire: An investigation of adults with Asperger syndrome or high-functioning autism, and normal sex differences. *Journal of Autism and Developmental Disorders*, 33, 509-516.

Howlin, P. and Moore, A. (1997). Diagnosis in autism a survey of over 1200 patients in the UK. *Autism*, 1, 135-162.

Howlin, P., Goode, S., Hutton, J., and Rutter, M. (2004). Adult outcome for children with autism. *Journal of Child Psychology and Psychiatry*, 45, 212-229.

Howlin, P., Mawhood, L. and Rutter, M. (2000). Autism and developmental receptive language disorder—a follow-up comparison in early adult life. II: Social behavioural, and psychiatric outcomes. *Journal of Child Psychology and Psychiatry and Allied Disciplines*, 41, 561-578.

Kalyva, E. (2011). *Autism: Educational and therapeutic approaches.* London: Sage.

Kalyva, E. (2012). Diagnosing and living with autism spectrum disorders in adulthood. In: C. E. Richardson and R. A. Wood (Eds.), *Autism Spectrum Disorders: New research* (pp. 169-178). Hauppage, NY: Nova Science Publishers.

Kalyva, E. (2013). Collaboration between parents of children with autism spectrum disorders and mental health professionals. In: M. Fitzerald (Ed.), *Recent advances in autism spectrum disorders - Volume I* (pp. 521-562). Prague: Intechopen.

Kalyva, E. and Avramidis, E. (2005). Improving communication between children with autism and their peers through the 'circle of friends'. *Journal of Applied Research in Intellectual Disabilities*, 18, 253-261.

Miles, M. B. and Huberman, A. M. (1994). *Qualitative data analysis* (2nd ed.). London: Sage Ltd.

Orsmond, G. I., Krauss, M. W. and Seltzer, M. M. (2004). Peer relationships and social and recreational activities among adolescents and adults with autism. *Journal of Autism and Developmental Disorders*, 34, 245-256.

Padgett, D. K. (1998). *Qualitative methods in social work research: Challenges and rewards.* Thousand Oaks, CA: Sage Publications.

Papageorgiou, V. and Kalyva, E. (2010). Self-reported needs and expectations of parents of children with autism spectrum disorders who participate in support groups. *Research in Autism Spectrum Disorders*, 4, 653-660.

Patton, M. Q. (2002). *Qualitative research and evaluation methods.* Thousand Oaks, CA: Sage Publications.

Seltzer, M. M., Krauss, M. W., Shattuck, P., Orsmond, G. I., Swe, A., and Lord, C. (2003). Changes in the symptoms of autism in adolescence and adulthood. *Journal of Autism and Developmental Disorders*, 33, 565-581.

Stokes, M., Newton, N. and Kaur, A. (2007). Stalking, and social and romantic functioning among adolescents and adults with autism spectrum disorder. *Journal of Autism and Developmental Disorders*, 37, 1969-1986.

In: Autism Spectrum Disorders
Editor: Arlene Valdez

ISBN: 978-1-63482-547-4

Chapter 5

The Effect of Group Cognitive Behavior Therapy on Adults with High-Functioning Autism Spectrum Disorder

***Yuko Furuhashi*[1*] *and Shusuke Furuhashi*[2]**
[1] Health Care Center, Shizuoka University, Japan
[2] Clinic of Oji plant, the National Printing Bureau, Japan

Abstract

Autism spectrum disorder (ASD) is a neurodevelopmental condition marked by impairment of social interaction, social communication and restricted and repetitive stereotyped patterns of behavior, interests and activities (American Psychiatric Association, 2000). ASD symptoms cause impairment across many functioning areas and are present early in life. Individuals with ASD are vulnerable to a lot of psychiatric and neurological disorders such as depression, epilepsy, sleep disorder, anxiety disorder, and obsessive compulsive disorder. In addition, hyper- or hyposensitivity to pain, touch, movement, sound, smell, and light is often reported (Minshew and Hobson, 2008). Recent reports suggest that adults with ASD are unable to understand their own mental states, which could lead to difficulties in emotional regulation. As a result of these

---

[*] Corresponding author: Yuko Furuhashi, email: furuhashi.yuko@shizuoka.ac.jp.

psychiatric and neurological difficulties, quality of life is often impaired in adults with ASD (Jeannes-Coussens at al., 2006). Various treatments have been developed to alleviate comorbid symptoms in adults with ASD. Psychological methods designed to treat children with ASD are difficult to adapt to adult patients with ASD because they either involve parental participation or are too time-consuming. However, some studies have reported the efficacy of cognitive behavior therapy (CBT) in improving emotional regulation among adults with ASD. In addition, group settings enable social interaction and sharing experiences with others, which reduces social isolation. Group CBT is additionally beneficial in terms of increasing specific skills and minimizing dropout. This review evaluates the evidence for the group CBT in adults with high functioning ASD.

1. Introduction

Autism spectrum disorder (ASD) is characterized by significant impairment in social interaction, verbal and nonverbal communication deficits, and restricted and repetitive interests and behaviors (APA, 2000). These symptoms range in severity from mild to severe and usually persist throughout the lifespan. The ASD label replaces former subtypes, including autism, pervasive developmental disorder-not otherwise specified (PDD-NOS), and Asperger's syndrome (AS) (APA, 2000). While many individuals with autism have intact or elevated intellectual abilities, non-social neurocognitive impairments have also been observed in such domains regarding speed of processing (Mayes and Calhoun 2007), aspects of working memory (Williams et al., 2005), planning (Hughes et al., 1994), and executive functioning (Oznoff, 1994). In addition, social cognitive impairments have been observed in many domains in autism, and include deficits in perspective taking (Mizuno et al., 2011), theory of mind (Baron-Cohen, 1990), emotion perception and management (Samson et al., 2012), and social context appraisal abilities (Wang et al., 2006). This constellation of social and non-social information processing deficits significantly limits the ability of individuals with high-functioning ASD to adapt and succeed in adult life in spite of normal intellectual abilities. Furthermore, it was shown that adults with ASD, including those with normal IQ, are at disadvantage with regard to employment, academic performance, social relationships, mental health, and quality of life (Howlin et al., 2004).

The prevalence of ASD has been examined in several studies, and the estimated prevalence of ASD diagnosis in children has been markedly rising in recent years. This represents a more-than-threefold increase from previously published figures, which estimated the prevalence of autism at approximately 5 per 10,000 (Fombonne, 2009). However, the results of an additional study reported that ASD affected 1 to 2.5% of children in the general population (Kim et al., 2011). While there are methodological differences between various prevalence studies, the rising prevalence of ASD has been well-documented across Western countries, including Europe, Australia, and the USA (Yeargin-Allsopp et al., 2003, Williams 2006, Kogan et al., 2009).

Increasing attention has been recently given to concomitant psychiatric conditions in patients with ASD. It is now known that individuals with ASD are vulnerable to a number of various psychiatric and neurological disorders such as depression, epilepsy, sleep disorder, anxiety disorder, and obsessive compulsive disorder. Poor social interaction skills represent the primary source of impairment in ASD, regardless of the individual's intelligence or language ability (Carter et al., 2009). The social disability that characterizes ASD does not diminish during childhood or adolescence, although it may be felt more acutely in adolescence (Tse et al., 2007).

Large-scale epidemiological data on the prevalence of co-occurring anxiety disorders are not available, however, a recent comprehensive review found estimates of impairing anxiety in children with ASD ranging from 11 % to 84 % (White et al., 2009).

The rate of mood and anxiety problems is significantly higher in children (Kim et al., 2000), adolescents (Barnhill, 2001) and adults (Ghaziuddin et al., 1998) with high-functioning ASD compared with that in the general population. Depression is possibly the most common psychiatric disorder found in people with ASD, and there has been some suggestion that individuals with high-functioning ASD may be particularly affected (Ghaziuddin, 2005).

In addition, hypersensitivity or hyposensitivity to pain, touch, movement, sound, smell, and light are often reported (Minshew and Hobson, 2008). Recent reports suggest that adults with ASD are unable to understand their own mental states, which could lead to difficulties in emotional regulation. As a result of these psychiatric and neurological difficulties, quality of life is often impaired in adults with ASD (Jeannes-Coussens et al., 2006).

As patients with ASD have emerged in clinical practice during the last decade, there is an urgent need to identify suitable treatment options. Treatments for ASD that families pursue include behavioral, educational, medical, allied health, and complementary approaches. Individual goals for treatment vary for different patients and may include combinations of therapies. While advances have been made in early detection and intervention approaches that attempt to limit the impact of ASD on individual and their families, few efforts have been dedicated to advancing the treatment of adults with ASD (Fitzpatric et al., 2013). In addition, psychological methods designed to treat children with ASD are difficult to adapt for use in adult patients with ASD because they either involve parental participation or are too time-consuming.

There is an urgent for the development of effective interventions designed to address core cognitive deficits in adults with ASD. Neurocognitive and social-cognitive impairments have a significant impact on social, vocational, and academic functioning as well as quality of life. Cognitive rehabilitation interventions offer a significant promise for remediating the broad social and non-social cognitive impairments associated with ASD. Cognitive rehabilitation represents a potentially effective approach for the remediation of information processing impairments in individuals with high-functioning ASD. Although antidepressants are widely used in patients with ASD, few corresponding efficacy data exist. In contrast, cognitive behavioral therapy (CBT) has shown promising results (Wood et al., 2009) and is safe and acceptable to families. Within the general population, CBT is the most widely researched and endorsed psychological intervention (James et al. 2005). CBT is a form of psychotherapy originally developed for the treatment of depression in the general population. The results of many studies have demonstrated that CBT is an effective treatment for anxiety and depression in typically developing children, adolescents, and adults (Compton et al., 2004, Klein et al., 2005). The defining feature of CBT is its mechanism of action for clinical improvement, which involves a change in cognition such that dysfunctional cognitive structures are corrected. Furthermore, the need for structure and predictability makes CBT an attractive treatment option for patients with ASD (Gaus et al., 2011). In addition, psycho-education on ASD and related psychiatric symptoms as well as social training are recommended as part of CBT (Gerhardt et al., 2010). There has been a growing interest in developing CBT for patients with ASD who continue to experience distress and functional interference due to persistent symptoms. Although CBT has become a widely practiced and empirically supported psychotherapeutic approach, it has only been advocated for use in the treatment of ASD in the past decade. There have been several recent reviews on the early empirical research on CBT for patients with ASD. Some studies have reported the efficacy of CBT in improving emotional regulation among adults with ASD, however, most of the literature on ASD focuses on children and adolescents. Unfortunately, comprehensive approaches designed to address the core neurocognitive and social-cognitive impairments in adults with ASD have yet to be developed. Furthermore, there is undoubtedly a need for the development of treatment options for adult psychiatric patients with ASD.

This article provides an update on the impact of group CBT for adults with high-functioning ASD. Although this is not a systematic review, published studies have been selected following a detailed search on Medline. The publications that are reviewed here were selected studies of group CBT for adults with high-functioning ASD. Therefore, the current review evaluates the literature using a comprehensively focused framework.

2. Methods

2.1. Search Procedure

An electronic search of databases was conducted through an academic search engine, MEDLINE.

Terms were entered for searching in the titles and abstracts of articles. Three search sets were used. The first search set pertained to autism and used the terms "autism spectrum disorder (ASD)" or "high-functioning ASD" or "pervasive developmental disorder -not otherwise specified (PDD-NOS)" or "Asperger's syndrome (AS)". The second search set pertained to cognitive behavior therapy (CBT) and used the terms "cognitive behavior therapy" or "group cognitive behavior therapy". The final search set pertained to adults and used the terms "adult" or "adulthood". The three search sets were linked with the instruction "AND".

2.2. Inclusion Criteria

The search sets included all publications from January 2000 to July 2014. The search was limited to publications that appeared in journals written in English and excluded dissertation abstracts. The search produced 33 publications. The abstracts from these publications were then reviewed to ensure that the studies investigated group CBT or ASD. We excluded case reports, reviews, book chapters, and studies which individual CBT were performed. In addition, we excluded studies with sample sizes less than three and those in which the mean age of the subjects was under 18 years. A total of seven studies met the criteria for inclusion in this review.

Table 1. Characteristic of group CBT trials in adults with ASD

study	n	mean age	study design	study duration	outcome measure
Palmen et al. 2011	12	20.75	pre-post	6 month 15+4 sessions	need for leisure support engagement in leisure activities
Weiss and Lunsky 2010	3	about45 (30-mid50)	pre-post	12 sessions, weekly	BAI, BDI-Ⅱ
Eack et al. 2013	14	25.29 (SD=5.72)	pre-post	18 month 45 sessions	CSQ-8, the MATRICS battery, the Cognitive Style and Social Cognition Eligibility Interview
Pugliese and White 2014	5	21.27 (18-23)	pre-post	9 sessions	SPSI-R, OQ45.2
McGillivray and Evert 2014	32	20.6 (SD=4.1)	RCT	9 sessions 2 hours, weekly	DASS, ATQ, ASSQ
Hesselmark et al. 2014	68	31.8 (SD=9.03)	RCT	36 sessions 3 hours, weekly	QOLI, SoC, RSES, AQ, ASRS, BDI, SCL, PCGI-S
Russel et al. 2013	46	26.9 (14-65)	RCT	up to 20 sessions 1 hour, weekly	YBOCS, CGI, OCI-R, BDI, BAI

BAI: Beck Anxiety Inventory, BDI-Ⅱ: Beck Depression Inventory-Ⅱ, WPP: Work Personality Profile, SIB-R: Scale of Independent Behavior Revised, OEI-R: Observational Emotional Inventory Revised, CSQ-8: Client Satisfaction Questionnaire-8, SPSI-R: Social Problem Solving Inventory-Revised, OQ 45.2: Outcome Questionnaire 45.2, DASS: Depression Anxiety Stress Scale, ATQ: Automatic Thoughts Questionnaire, ASSQ: Anxious Self-Statements Questionnaire, QOLI: Quality of Life Inventory, SoC: Sense of Coherence, RSES: Rosenberg Self-Esteem Scale, AQ: Autism Quotient, ASRS: Adult ADHD Self-Repot Scale, SCL: Symptom Checklist, PCGI-S: Patient Rated Clinical Global Improvement-Severity, YBOCS: Yale-Brown Obsessive Compulsive Scale, CGI: Clinical Global Impression, OCI-R: Obsessive Compulsive Inventory-Revised,

3. Results

3.1. Overview of Reviewed Studies

Table 1 provides an overview of the reviewed articles. Two of the seven studies were performed in the United States. Australia, Sweden, Canada, the United Kingdom, and the Netherlands each contributed one study.

Sample sizes ranged from N = 3 to N = 68. These studies can be divided into two groups according to the study setting, single-group CBT studies using a pre-post design, and randomized controlled trials (RCTs) of group CBT for adults with ASD.

3.2. Single-Group CBT

There are four published single-group CBT studies that used a pre-post design.

Palmen et al. (2011) examined the effectiveness of group CBT for high-functioning young adults living either at home or within an independent setting. A pre-test-post-test control group design was used. Participants were 12 high-functioning young adults with ASD. At the start of the program, participants were between 16 and 31 years of age (mean 20.75 years), and two of them were female. Two members of the treatment facility staff participated as program leaders and they led the sessions under supervision of Palmen. In general, each session consisted of seven components: 1) a warming-up in which participants could discuss leisure events that had occurred in the previous session; 2) an evaluation of participant's homework whereby feedback was given by the other participants and /or program leader and problems in homework were discussed; 3) an introduction of the session's topic, in which the importance of the topic was discussed and , in the case of leisure skills , the components of the skills were analyzed, discussed and visualized; 4) a short break; 5) behavioral practice and feedback, in which skills were practiced using role-play or real life exercises; 6) an instruction in homework for the next session, in which an appointment was made with each participant by the program leader for delivering support by mail or telephone; 7) a brief evaluation of the content of the session. They reported that an outpatient group training program, consisting of client-supported strategies and cognitive behavioral components, was effective in improving the leisure lifestyle of high-functioning young adults with ASD.

Weiss and Lunsky (2010) described the use of a published and empirically supported manualized CBT treatment for mood and anxiety disorders, referred to as Mind Over Mood (Greenberger and Padesky, 1995), for adult with ASD. They conducted CBT, which was provided over 12 weekly one hour sessions based on the structure and information provided in the Mind Over Mood workbook (Padesky and Greenberger, 1995) and the Mind Over Mood Clinicians Guide (Greenberger and Padesky, 1995). Participants were three high-functioning adults with ASD whose ages ranged from 30 to 60 years. Each participant purchased a copy of the book and was assigned homework that included reading and completing a specific chapter after each session. Each session consisted of the same structure: setting the agenda, check in, homework review, new content, assigning homework and feedback. Weiss and Lunsky reported that an outpatient group training program was effective in improving mood and anxiety in high-functioning adults with ASD. In addition, Weiss and Lunsky reported that all their patients appreciated the small size of the group and the individual attention they received from the therapists and co-participants regarding specific situations, which was likely more time intensive than that in a typical group. Interestingly, patients reported that they could relate to the case vignette provided in the workbook and did not want to replace these vignettes with individuals with ASD. They appreciated the charts in the book but found it more helpful to redesign the tables in a computer format, so that they would be more individualized. The 12-week group showed some promise in addressing symptoms of anxiety or depression. In addition, study results suggested that there were a number of advantages to providing CBT to adults with ASD within a group that is composed of other individuals with ASD.

Eack et al. (2013) reported that 12 adults with ASD and an average age of 25.29 years enrolled in a feasibility study of Cognitive Enhanced Therapy (CET). CET integrates 60 hours of computer-based neurocognitive training in attention, memory, and problem-solving with a structured 45-session social-cognitive group curriculum designed to facilitate the achievement of adult social-cognitive milestones, particularly perspective-taking and social context appraisal. Neurocognitive training exercises are all computer based and are divided into three modules: attention, memory, and problem-solving. After several months of neurocognitive training in attention, 6-8 participants (3-4 pairs) come together to form a social-cognitive group. Through the use of in vivo cognitive exercises and psycho-education, the weekly 1.5 hour social-cognitive group sessions provide a rich secondary socialization experience that targets a broad, theoretically-driven array of social-cognitive abilities ranging from abstracting the gist from spontaneous, unrehearsed social interactions to understanding the perspectives of others, accurately appraising novel social contexts, and managing emotions. Social-cognitive group sessions are designed to make effective use of the group context to provide secondary socialization opportunities to participants, which is a fundamental avenue for higher-order social-cognitive development. Eack et al. (2013) reported that CET was satisfying to participants with high treatment attendance and retention. Effects on cognitive deficits and social behavior were large and significant. Their results suggested that CET was a feasible and effective intervention for remediating the social and non-social cognitive impairments in adults with ASD.

Pugliese and White (2014) conducted the pre-to post-treatment single subject. This study adapted and piloted a group-based cognitive-behavioral intervention program. Problem Solving Skills: 101 (PSS: 101), to teach effective problem solving abilities to college students with ASD. Five students with ASD participated in this study. All participants were males and between 18 and 23 years of age. The groups were facilitated by two clinical psychologists. Treatment integrity was assessed via ratings jointly completed by the therapists at the end of each treatment session. Specific components intended for every session included posting of the group agenda, discussing homework assignments, and completing goals during each session. During the beginning of PSS: 101, students selected a problem they wished to work on for the remainder of the program. Problem Solving Skills: 101 (PSS: 101) consisted of nine sessions. The purpose of the first session was to provide an overview of PSS: 101 and to establish a positive therapeutic relationship. Sessions two through four focused on the importance of a positive problem orientation in relation to problem solving, such as viewing problems as challenges rather than threats (D'Zurilla and Nezu, 2007). Sessions five through eight focused on practicing discrete skills of the problem solving process, such as problem definition and formulation, using brainstorming techniques to generate alternative solutions to maximize the likelihood of an effective solution, decision making, and solution implementation including self-monitoring and self-evaluation of the solution outcome (D'Zurilla and Nezu, 2007). In session nine, students evaluated their attempts to implement their chosen solution and re-worked their solution plans. Pugliese reported that four of the five participants completed at least eight of the nine sessions and that between-session assignments were generally completed indicating a high level of treatment adherence. In addition, all of the participants indicated that they liked the PSS: 101 program and found it to be moderately helpful, and most were satisfied with the topics of the meetings. Most group members also indicated that they found group meetings to be the most helpful component of PSS: 101. Every participant indicated that they had a positive experience meeting others with ASD on the endpoint consumer satisfaction questionnaire. Specifically, participants stated that it was helpful to meet other students with ASD in order to have people in similar situations to talk with, to see that many of the group members share the same problems, and to learn how others with ASD solve their problems.

These four single-group studies showed that group CBT for adults with ASD was effective. In spite of some positive findings from these single-group studies, the relatively small number of participants and lack of a randomly assigned comparison group limit the generalization of the findings, as any of the noted improvements could still be attributable to individual sample characteristics.

3.3. Randomized Controlled Trials of Group CBT

There are three studies using randomized controlled trials (RCT) of group CBT for those with high-functioning ASD.

McGillivray and Evert (2014) examined the efficacy of group-delivered CBT on the reduction of symptoms of depression, anxiety and stress in young adults with ASD. Participants were forty two young adults with ASD aged 15-25 years, with a mean age of 20.6 years. The participants were allocated either to a treatment group (N = 26) or a wait-list control group (N = 16) according to alternating order of enrolment. There were no group differences in gender, educational level, employment status, or in the population that lived with their parents. McGillivray and Evert utilized a quasi-experimental design. To make comparisons between those allocated to the group intervention program and the individuals allocated to a wait-list. The group intervention program was conducted over 9 weeks and each session was approximately 2 hours in duration. At the outset, the focus of the program was to identify the nature of the events that participants found stressful as well as the extent to which these events were related to the interactions of all participants with others. The role of emotions and awareness of feelings was then highlighted. McGillivray and Evert reported that a CBT-based group intervention program showed promise in assisting the reduction of negative symptoms in young adults with ASD. Furthermore, they reported that the intervention program appeared to have a positive effect in terms of a reduction of symptoms of depressed mood and stress in comparison to those on the wait-list.

Hesselmark et al. (2014) performed a RCT that compared a CBT group with a recreational activity group. A total of 68 adults with high-functioning ASD were allocated randomly to the CBT group or a recreational activity group. The mean age of participants at recruitment was 31.8 years. Participants received 36 sessions of group CBT or recreational activity per week. The CBT intervention consisted of five elements: 1) structure; 2) group setting; 3) psycho-education; 4) social training; and 5) cognitive behavioral techniques. In addition, the treatment was divided into three thematic modules: a) self-esteem and ASD awareness; b) social contacts and everyday life; c) psychological and physical health. Each session followed a strict agenda: 1) introduction and presentation of the agenda of the day; 2) review of homework assignments from the previous session; 3) psycho-educatinal lecture and discussions on the session topic; 4) coffee break with buns or sandwiches and social interaction; 5) relaxation or mindfulness; 6) discussion and exercises on the session topic; 7) distribution of homework; 8) evaluation and end of session. On the other hand, the purpose of the recreational activity interaction was to facilitate social interactions and break social isolation. This intervention relied on structure and group setting only. As outcome measures, they adopted the Quality of Life Inventory (QOLI; Frisch et al.,1992), the Rosenberg Self-Esteem Scale (RSES; Rosenberg, 1962), Sense of Coherence scale (SoC; Antonovsky, 1993), the Beck Depression Inventory (BDI; Beck et al., 1996), the Symptom Checklist 90 (SCL-90; Derogatis and Cleary, 1977), the Autism Quotient (AQ; Baron-Cohen et al., 2001), the Adult ADHD self-Repot Scale (ASRS; Kessler et al., 2005), the self-rated Clinical Global Impression Scale-Severity (CGI-S) and the Clinical Global Impression Scale-Improvement (CGI-I; Guy, 1976). They followed up six-month and one year. This study successfully developed and compared two group interventions for adults with ASD. The group CBT and group recreational activity interventions were equally beneficial to participants in increasing their quality of life. Psychiatric symptoms and self-esteem were not affected by either intervention. The CBT participants reported a better sense of well-being, and a greater understanding of their own difficulties compared with that in participants in the recreational activity intervention.

Russell et al. (2013) randomized forty six patients with obsessive compulsive disorder (OCD) to receive up to 20 sessions of a CBT intervention or an anxiety management (AM), intervention, which was considered to be a plausible control treatment. Participants were individuals with a confirmed diagnosis of an ASD and comorbid OCD aged between 14 and 65 years.

Standard CBT for OCD was adapted by 1) ensuring the building blocks for treatment were in place; 2) educational sessions about understanding and rating anxiety, if required, were provided before moving on to present the rationale for treatment; 3) visual tools and concrete/special interest related analogies were used to convey psychological concepts; 4) a structured and therapist-directed approach to sessional and homework content was taken. The CBT treatment was predominantly exposure and response prevention (ERP) based, and was conducted in the usual hierarchal fashion both in sessions and as homework. The control or comparison treatment was specified as anxiety management (AM) to ensure that any treatment effects were solely due to the adapted CBT for OCD rather than therapist contact, psycho-education about anxiety, or general anxiety reduction techniques. The AM manual comprised eight modules, which were adapted for ASD by including visual aids or concrete examples. Symptoms were rated by assessors blind to treatment group prior to commencing treatment, and at 1, 3, 6, and 12-month follow up. Assessors were all trained clinicians experienced in administering the Yale-Brown Obsessive Compulsive Scale (YBOCS) and interviewing people with ASD. The results of this study suggested that CBT was effective for comorbid OCD in adults with ASD. AM was also effective in bringing about a reduction in OCD symptoms in people with ASD, particularly those with milder symptoms. These results were considered to be highly encouraging and supportive of the efficacy of CBT for OCD.

3.4. Summary of Evidence for Group CBT

The results of these studies indicated that group CBT interventions were effective for adults with high-functioning ASD. Compared to the randomized studies, the single-group CBT studies produced more effective results. However, Tarrier and Wykes (2004) pointed out that studies of CBT for psychosis with poorer methodology often overestimate the benefits of treatment. Non-blind assessments are associated with exaggerated effects, making randomized studies more reliable. In addition, the large and strict RCTs might suggest group CBT for ASD can improve social behavior and general symptoms.

While both single-group CBT and randomized controlled CBT studies described different in various factors such as duration of the interventions, the number of sessions, the comparison treatment, and outcomes post-intervention and follow-up, a number of common findings emerged. CBT appears to be particularly effective as an adjunct to medication in helping patients with the psychopathology of ASD. Furthermore, the nonspecific therapy may be more potent in these groups, as they often socially isolated and lack support.

4. Discussion

4.1. Review Summary

There are only a few studies that have examined the efficacy of group CBT in treating the mental health problems of adults with high-functioning ASD. In addition, several case studies of adults with high-functioning ASD have suggested that CBT can also benefit for this population (Cardaciotto and Herbertl, 2004, Hare, 1997).

Indeed, there are only three RCTs which have explored the use of CBT in this population. Most of the literature on ASD focuses on children and adolescents. However, ASD leads to lifelong disabilities and services are gradually developing for adults with ASD.

This review suggested that most of the studies of group CBT for adults with high-functioning ASD showed various benefits at the end of treatment, however, the benefits tended to be lost after follow-up in several studies.

Several of the publications on group CBT for high-functioning ASD in this review investigated only a cohort of patients at the beginning and end of treatment (Weiss and Lunsky, 2010, Eack et al., 2013, Pugliese and White, 2014). These studies provided evidence for the feasibility and acceptability of this form of group CBT treatment. Most of the participants in those studies reported that they could talk about their symptoms with group members after the first or second sessions, and there were no reports of problems in facilitating the groups.

Although there is limited empirical support for the use of CBT in the treatment of adults with high-functioning ASD, there is a growing literature based on case studies and a few small, uncontrolled intervention studies suggesting that CBT can be used effectively to treat social skills impairments, anxiety, and depression in this population.

Based on the results of this review, it would seem that group CBT for adults with high-functioning ASD may represent a potentially effective treatment. Nevertheless, CBT should be considered as a component of a widespread treatment combination that also includes social interventions and medications. Unfortunately, CBT may be limited by a low level of service delivery, as there are simply not enough trained therapists to cover the potential patient base. In addition, more research into the functioning elements of CBT will be required.

The results of this review indicated that anxiety and depressive mood were improved in most of the participants. For example, Lui (2013) reported that significant improvements were shown in WPP for workplace social behaviors, SIB-R for social communication skills, and OEI-R for emotional control. However, these uncontrolled studies show the difficulty in trying to identify an outcome measure that can represent a change in what is essentially a highly variable experience. According to the results of RCTs conducted by Hesselmark et al. (2014) and Russell et al. (2013), group CBT can improve social behavior, OCD symptoms, and general symptoms. There is also evidence that it can reduce anxiety and increase coping strategies. The results of RCTs were mixed for improvements in self-esteem, distress, and anxiety. In addition, many positive results were reduced when comparing CBT to an active treatment control such as AM. While these studies suggest that group CBT appears to be particularly effective, additional research will be required to refine CBT in terms of identifying the most effective components and the best methods for delivery. A more rigorous research design using methodologically strict randomized clinical trials that include comparisons of treatments and independent evaluators will also be required to evaluate treatment efficacy.

4.2. Implication for CBT for ASD in Clinical Practice

1) Pertinent Components and Characteristics of CBT for Patients with ASD

Some aspects of the CBT program were noted to be particularly helpful for patients with ASD. Patients appreciated the predictability of the intervention, in that each session was structured with an agenda, the discussions were based on what they had read in the book and questions posed to each of them followed the structure in the manual. Structure is even more important for patients with ASD. As these patients with ASD show deficits in executive functioning that affect planning, motivation, organizing, and prioritizing. These deficits impose inflexibility in problem-solving, and impair time-perception and management. Provision of external structure is important

group of treatment approaches collectively referred to as cognitive rehabilitation has emerged in other disorders, and may represent potentially effective non-pharmacologic interventions for the core information processing deficits associated with adults with ASD.

The group therapy component includes more frequent group sessions of longer duration in order to teach additional social skills and allow for a greater emphasis on practice within the group. In addition, all the key CBT factors can be provided within a group format, which may provide additional therapeutic opportunities. Group treatment offers several advantages over individual therapy. For example, the group setting can provide a forum to test out new beliefs and coping strategies as well as facilitate other group processes that can enhance wellbeing, such as the chance to help others. Furthermore, it may be more cost-effective to offer treatment in groups, given the recommendation for experienced therapists to implement CBT for ASD.

An individual with ASD may feel like an outsider in a group of typically developing peers, which can induce feeling of isolation that often manifest as anxiety and depressive mood. On the other hand, the results of several studies examining the characteristics of children with ASD have demonstrated significant decreases in anxiety symptoms following participation in the manualized group CBT intervention (Reaven et al. 2009, Chalfant et al. 2007, Sofronoff et al. 2005). These results are promising, especially given the high rates of comorbidity between ASD and anxiety (Attood 2005). In addition, these results also provide initial support for the feasibility of implementing CBT in a group context for participants with ASD.

Treatment delivered in a group context may not only ease feelings of isolation that are often common for these families but also provide a natural opportunity for growth in positive social interactions. Therefore, groups may help to reduce anxiety through the presentation of a normative view of ASD. Most group members also indicated that they found group meetings to be the most helpful component of the therapy. Every participant indicated that they had a positive experience meeting others with ASD on the end-point questionnaire. Further, participants with ASD stated that it was helpful to meet other patients with ASD in order to have people in similar situations to talk with, to see that many of the group members share the same problems, and to learn how others with ASD solve their problems. The group setting may have helped normalize their problems in such an environment. While there are some pragmatic considerations, it is believed that a group modality offers some benefits relative to an individual intervention for various reasons. In spite of the diverse symptomatology of ASD, many individuals in the group had similar problems in their wider environments and group therapy created a forum for participants to offer advice, strategies, and insight to other group members. Whereas an individual with ASD may feel like an outsider in a group of typically developing peers, the group therapy modality provides the opportunity to feel accepted and understood by a group of peers who struggle with the same disorder and offers the chance to practice problem solving skills in a relatively naturalistic, but safe and supportive environment. Thus, group therapy can provide a sense of being normal, and understood as well as provide a safe space to talk about an isolated experience.

Group members may be more likely to be sympathetic and understanding of behaviors associated with ASD, which typically developing individuals may find off-putting. Group therapy also afforded the opportunity for role-playing, where observers provided constructive feedback on the problem solving processes of other individuals.

4.3. Implications for Future Research

Although there is limited empirical support for the use of cognitive behavioral techniques in the treatment of adults with high-functioning ASD, there is a growing literature based on case reports and some small, uncontrolled intervention studies suggesting that CBT can be used effectively to treat social skill impairments, anxiety, and depression in adults with ASD.

It is difficult for adults with high-functioning ASD in terms of adults to live. The transition into adulthood is often a challenging time for relatively young people with ASD. The social impairments inherent in high-functioning autism interfere with the processes of relationship building, occupational functioning, and participating and integrating into the community, all of which are aspects of social functioning that take on a larger role during the transition to adulthood. For many adults with ASD, handling these new social demands can be difficult. Recognition of these challenges has contributed to the development of treatments for adults with ASD that aim to increase functioning by focusing on selected social skills, which in turn may improve social cognition and social functioning. However, there are few evidence-based interventions for adults with ASD that apply to either the social skills or cognition approaches.

Measuring change over the course of social interventions remains ambiguous in terms of identifying which are the most informative variables (Cunningham 2013). Previous adult interventions have quantified social skills and cognition over time using a variety of techniques and measures with mixed success. Another approach to measuring social change is through the use of social cognition performance measures. Performance measures are recorded while participants engage in social tasks and the accuracy of the response is quantified. In this study, improvements were found on measures of emotional recognition, however, other measures of theory of mind and conventional skills did not show a change after the intervention (Turner-Brown et al., 2008). Overall, the pervious literature regarding patients with high functioning ASD has demonstrated that targeted interventions can improve social skills and social cognition. However, the majority of these interventions have been social skills-based and group-based, which may limit the amount of social skills practice and the amount of time spent interacting with others outside the autism spectrum. These interventions probable also have been somewhat limited by imagination of the participants, and such limitations have been noted as deficient in this population (Herrera et al., 2008). This lack of real-world training may hinder the generalization of treatment effects. Less is known about the potential changes in social skills and social cognition when conducted in an individual real-time simulation of authentic social interactions with neurotypical adults.

An additional consideration for further research is the range of outcomes. There is a need for a robust measure of relapse, which can be applied consistently across studies. The lack of effect on relapse rates can be understood in this context. It is clear that further research will be required in order to better understand the effect of CBT based on the different stages of presenting symptoms. In patients prone to relapse and recovery, the use of CBT to reduce relapse should be investigated. In part, the answers to these questions may result in a better understanding of the process of change in treatment. For example, OCD and ASD are frequently comorbid (Abramson et al., 2005), and there is evidence to suggest that the active ingredient of a CBT protocol for individuals with OCD should be qualitatively different from interventions addressing generalized and social anxiety symptoms (Barrett et al., 2005). Research also needs to be conducted in order to determine if this is applicable for individuals with ASD who have comorbid OCD. Finally, additional research will also be required in order to refine the treatment in terms of identifying the most effective components and the best methods for delivery.

Conclusion

There is a growing population of adults with ASD seeking psychotherapy. This study addressed the shortage of treatment options for adults with high-functioning ASD. Preliminary evidence suggests that group CBT may be efficacious for adults with high-functioning ASD. As previously mentioned, future directions for CBT research include more robust and well-designed studies to determine the most effective components of CBT. In addition, studies will need to focus on a component analysis to evaluate the mechanisms by which change occurred, ultimately leading to more efficient or effective interventions for adults with high-functioning ASD. Furthermore, future CBT trials should consider extending the follow-up period for longer durations, which may provide additional information about the natural course of symptoms.

References

Abramson RK, Ravan SA, Wright HH, et al. (2005). The relationship between restrictive and repetitive behaviors in individuals with autism and obsessive compulsive symptoms in parents. *Child Psychiatry Hum Dev.* 36(2), 155-65..

American Psychiatric Association (2013). *Diagnostic and Statistical Manual of Mental Disorders* - V. Washington, DC, APA, 2013.

American Psychiatric Association (1994). *Diagnostic and Statistical Manual of Mental Disorders* (DSM VI), Washington DC, APA, 1994.

Anderson S, Morris J (2006). Cognitive behavior therapy for people with Asperger syndrome. *Behavioral and Cognitive Psychotherapy* 34, 293-303.

Antonovsky A (1993). The structure and properties of the Sense of Coherence Scale. *Social Science and Medicine* 36 (6), 725-733.

Attwood T (2005). Cognitive behavioral therapy for children and adults with Asperger's syndrome. *Behavior Change* 21, 147-161.

Barnhill T (2002). Asperger Syndrome: An Overview of Characteristics. *Focus Autism Other Developmental Disability* 17 (3), 132-137.

Bauminger N (2002). The facilitation of social emotional understanding and social interaction in high-functioning children with autism: intervention outcomes. *Journal of Autism and Developmental Disorders* 32, 283-298.

Baron-Cohen S (1990). Autism: A specific cognitive disorder of mind-blindness. *International Review of Psychiatry* 2 (1), 81-90.

Baron-Cohen S, Wheelwright S, Skinner R, et al. (2001). The autism-spectrum quotient (AQ): evidence from Asperger syndrome/high-functioning autism, males and females, scientists and mathematicians. *Journal of Autism and Developmental Disorders* 31 (1), 5-17.

Barrett P, Farrell L, Dadds M, et al. (2005). Cognitive-behavioral family treatment of childhood obsessive compulsive disorder: long-term follow-up and predictors of outcome. *Journal of the American Academy of Child and Adolescent Psychiatry* 44, 1005-1014.

Beck AT, Steer RA, Ball R, et al. (1996). Comparison of Beck Depression Inventories I A and II in psychiatric outpatients, *Journal of Personality Assessment* 67(3), 588-597.

Cardaciotto L and Herbert JD (2004). Cognitive behavior therapy for social anxiety disorder in the context of Asperger's syndrome: A single-subject report. *Cognitive and Behavioral Practice* 11, 75-81.

Carter AS, Black DO, Tewani S, et al. (2007). Sex differences in toddlers with autism spectrum disorders. *Journal of Autism and Developmental Disorders* 37(1), 86-97.

Chadwick P, Sambrooke S, Rasch S, et al. (2000). Challenging the omnipotence of voices: group cognitive behavior therapy for voices. *Behaviour Research and Therapy* 38, 993-1003.

Chalfant AM, Rapee R, Carroll L (2007). Treating anxiety disorders in children with high functioning autism spectrum disorders: a controlled trial. *Journal of Autism and Developmental Disorders* 37, 1842-1857.

Compton SN, March JS, Brent D, et al. (2004). Cognitive behavioral psychotherapy for anxiety and depressive disorders in children and adolescents: An evidence based medicine review. *Journal of the American Academy of Child and Adolescent Psychiatry* 43 (8), 930-959.

Derogatis LB, Cleary PA (1977). Confirmation of the dimensional structure of the SCL-90: a study in construct validation. *Journal of Clinical Psychology* 33(4), 981-990.

D'Zurilla TJ, Nezu AM (2007). *Problem-solving therapy: A positive approach to clinical intervention* (3rd ed). New York, Springer.

Eack MS, Greenwald DP, Hogarty SS, et al. (2013). Cognitive Enhancement Therapy for Adults with Autism Spectrum Disorder: Results of an 18-month Feasibility Study. *Journal of Autism and Developmental Disorders* 43, 2866-2877.

Fitzpatrick P[1], Diorio R, Richardson MJ, et al. (2013). Dynamical methods for evaluating the time-dependent unfolding of social coordination in children with autism. *Frontiers in Integrative Neuroscience 7*, 1-13.

Frisch MB, Cornell J, Villanueva M et al. (1992). Clinical validation of the Quality of Life Inventory. A measure of life satisfaction for use in treatment planning and outcome assessment. *Psychological Assessment* 4(1), 92-101.

Fombonne E (2009). Epidemiology of pervasive developmental disorders. *Pediatric Research* 65, 591-598.

Gaus VL (2011). Cognitive behavioural therapy for adults with autism spectrum disorder. *Advances in Mental Health and Intellectual Disabilities* 5(5), 15 - 25.

Gerhardt PF, Lainer I (2011). Addressing the Needs of Adolescents and Adults with Autism: A Crisis on the Horizon. *Journal of Contemporary Psychotherapy* 41, 37–45.

Ghaziuddin M (2005). A family history study of Asperger syndrome. *Journal of Autism and Developmental Disorders* 35(2), 177-82..

Ghaziuddin M, Weidmer-mikhail E, Ghaziuddin N (1998). Comorbidity of Asperger syndrome: a preliminary report. *Journal of Intellectual Disability Research* 42, 279-283.

Greenberger D, Padesky CA (1995). *Mind over mood: Change how you feel by changing the way you think.* New York, Guilford Press.

Guy W (1976). The Clinical Global Impressions Scale. *ECDEU Assessment Manual for Psychopharmacology Revised*, Rockville. MD: National Institute of Mental Health, 218-222.

Hara DJ (1997). The use of cognitive-behavioral therapy with people with Asperger syndrome: A case study. *Autism* 1 (2), 215-225.

Herrera G[1], Alcantud F, Jordan R, et al. (2008). Development of symbolic play through the use of virtual reality tools in children with autistic spectrum disorders: two case studies. *See comment in PubMed Commons belowAutism.*12 (2), 143-157.

Hesselmark E, Plenty S, Bejerot S (2013). Group cognitive behavioral therapy and group recreational activity for adults with autism spectrum disorders: A preliminary randomized controlled trial. *Autism* 18 (6), 672-683.

Howlin P, Goode S, Rutter M (2004). Adult outcome for children with autism. *Journal of Child and Psychiatry* 45 (2), 212-229.

Hughes C[1], Russell J, Robbins TW (1994). Evidence for executive dysfunction in autism. *Neuropsychologia* 32 (4), 477-92.

Jennes-Coussens M[1], Magill-Evans J, Koning C (2006). The quality of life of young men with Asperger syndrome: a brief report. *Autism.* 2006 10 (4), 403-14..

James A, Soler A, Weatherall R (2005). Cognitive behavioural therapy for anxiety disorders in children and adolescents. *Cochrane Database of Systematic Reviews Issue 4 Art.* No: CD004690. DOI: 10.1002/14651858.CD004690.pub2..

Kessler RC, Adler L, Ames M, et al. (2005). The World Health Organization adult ADHD self-Report Scale (ASRs): a short screening scale for use in the general population. *Psychological Medicine* 35 (2), 245-256.

Kim JA, Szatmari P, Bryson SE, et al. (2000). The prevalence of anxiety and mood problems among children with autism and Asperger syndrome. *Autism* 4, 117-132.

Kim YS, Leventhal BL, Koh YJ, et al. (2011). Prevalence of autism spectrum disorders in a total population sample. *American Journal of Psychiatry* 168, 904-912.

Klin A, Pauls R, Schultz R, et al. (2005). Three diagnostic approaches to Asperger syndrome: Implications for research. *Journal of Autism and Developmental Disorders* 35, 221-231.

Kogen MD, Blumberg SJ, Schieve LA, et al. (2009). Prevalence of parent-reported diagnosis of autism spectrum disorder among children in the US, 2007. *Pediatrics* 124 (5), 1395-1403.

Lecomte T, Leclerc C, Wykes T, et al. (2008). Group cognitive behaviour therapy or social skills training for individuals with a first episode of psychosis? Results of a randomized controlled trial. *Journal of Nervous and Mental Disease* 196, 866-875.

Liu KPY, Wong D, Anthony CY, et al. (2013). Effectiveness of a Workplace Training Programme in Improving Social, Communication and Emotional Skills for Adults with Autism and Intellectual Disability in Hong Kong - A Pilot Study. *Occupational Therapy International* 20, 198-204.

Mayes SD, Calhoun SL (2007). Learning, attention, writing, and processing speed in typical children and children with ADHD, autism, anxiety, depression, and oppositional-defiant disorder. *Child Neuropsychology* 13(6), 469-93.

McGillivray JA, Evert HT (2014). Group Cognitive Behavioural Therapy Program Shows Potential in Reducing Symptoms of Depression and Stress among Young People with ASD. *Journal of Autism and Developmental Disorders* 44, 2041-2051.

Minshew NJ, Hobson JA (2008). Sensory sensitivities and performance on sensory perceptual tasks in high-functioning individuals with autism. *Journal Autism Developmental Disorders* 38(8), 1485-98.

Mizuno A, Liu Y, Williams DL, et al. (2011). The neural basis of deictic shifting in linguistic perspective-taking in high-functioning autism. *Brain* 134 (8), 2422-2435.

Newton E, landau S, Smith P, et al. (2005). Early psychological intervention for auditory hallucinations: An exploratory study of young people's voice group. *Journal of Nervous and Mental Disease* 193 (1), 58-61.

Ozonoff S, Strayer DL, McMahon WM, et al. (1994). Executive function abilities in autism and Tourette syndrome: an information processing approach. *Journal of Child Psychology and Psychiatry* 35 (6), 1015-32..

Palmen A, Didden R, Korzilius H (2011). An outpatient group training programme for improving leisure lifestyle in high-functioning young adults with ASD: A pilot study. *Development Neurorehabilitation* 14 (5), 297-309.

Padesky CA Greenberger D (1995). *Clinician's guide to mind over mood.* New York, Guilford Press.

Puglise CE, White SW (2014). Brief Report: Problem Solving Therapy in College Students with Autism Spectrum Disorders: Feasibility and Preliminary Efficacy. *Journal of Autism and Developmental Disorders* 44, 719-729.

Reaven J, Blakeley-Smith A, Culhane-Shelburne K, et al. (2012). Group cognitive behavior therapy for children with high-functioning autism spectrum disorders and anxiety: a randomized trial. *Journal of Child Psychology and Psychiatry and Allied Disciplines* 53, 410-419.

Rosenberg M (1962). The association between self-esteem and anxiety. *Journal of Psychiatric Research* 1, 135-152.

Russell AJ, Jassi A, Fullana MA, et al. (2013). Cognitive behavior therapy for comoebid obsessive-compulsive disorder in high-functioning autism spectrum disorders: a randomized controlled trail. *Depression and Anxiety* 30, 697-708.

Samon AC, Huber O, Gross JJ (2012). Emotion regulation in Asperger's syndrome and high-functioning autism. *Emotion* 12 (4), 659-665.

Sofronoff K, Attwood T (2003). A cognitive behavior therapy intervention for anxiety in children with Asperger's syndrome. *Good Autism Practice* 4, 2-8.

Sofronoff K, Attwood T, Hinton S (2005). A randomized controlled trial of a CBT intervention for anxiety in children with Asperger syndrome. *Journal of Child Psychology and Psychiatry* 46, 1152-1160.

Tarrier N, Wykes T (2004). Is there evidence that cognitive behaviour therapy is an effective treatment for schizophrenia? A cautions or cautionary tale? *Behaviour Research and Therapy* 42, 1377-1401.

Tse J, Strulovitch J, Tagalakis V, et al. (2007). Sosial skill treatment for adolescents with Asperger syndrome and high-functioning autism. *Journal of Autism and Developmental Disorders* 37 (10), 1960-1968.

Turner-Brown LM, Perry TD, et al. (2008). Dichter GS,Brief report: feasibility of social cognition and interaction training for adults with high functioning autism. *Journal of Autism and Developmental Disorders* 38 (9), 1777-1784.

Wang AT, Less SS, Sigman M, et al. (2006). Neural basis of irony comprehension in children with autism: the role of prosody and context. *Brain* 129 (4), 932-943.

Weiss JA, Lunsky Y (2010). Group Cognitive Behaviour Therapy for Adults with Asperger syndrome and anxiety or mood disorder: A case series. *Clinical Psychology and Psychiatry* 17, 438-446.

White SW, Oswald D, Ollendick T, et al. (2009). Anxiety in children and adolescents with autism spectrum disorders. *Clinical Psychology Review* 29 (3), 216-229.

Williams JH, Waiter GD, Gilchrist A, et al. (2006). Neural mechanisms of imitation and 'mirror neuron' functioning in autistic spectrum disorder. *Neuropsychologia* 44 (4), 610-21.

Wood JJ, Drahola A, Sze K, et al. (2009). Cognitive behavioral therapy for anxiety in children with autism spectrum disorders: a randomized controlled trail. *Journal of Child Psychology and Psychiatry and Allied Disciplines* 50, 224-234.

Yeargin-Allsopp M, Rice C, Karapurkar T, et al. (2003). Prevalence of autism in a US metropolitan area. *JAMA* 289(1), 49-55.

Abstract

Children with high-functioning autism spectrum disorder (HFASD) present with core deficits in social communication and restricted, repetitive, and stereotyped behaviors and interests that significantly impact their functioning and warrant comprehensive interventions. The knowledge and resources required to provide comprehensive interventions presents a particular challenge to treatment providers in school settings. The current chapter describes a systematic model of training and support provided to school professionals in order to guide and assist their implementation of a manualized comprehensive school-based intervention (schoolMAX) for 6-11 year old children with HFASD across the school year. The schoolMAX program was specifically designed to target the needs of children with HFASD within a school setting via social skills groups, therapeutic activities, face-voice emotion recognition instruction, individualized daily notes, and parent training. The implementation protocol consists of a three component process that includes 1) instruction, observation, planning, and practice; 2) treatment fidelity monitoring; and 3) consultative feedback. First, didactic instruction, observation, practice, and planning are used to build school staff knowledge and proficiency and to adapt the intervention to the participating school environment. Second, treatment fidelity is monitored throughout implementation by research clinicians to ensure the intervention protocol is conducted consistently and accurately. These research clinicians monitor fidelity while also providing ongoing modeling and support. Third, regular consultative feedback on provider proficiency is delivered to school staff by the senior research team. This feedback reviews ongoing intervention fidelity, problem-solves implementation issues, and evaluates student progress. Using data from the first year of a 4-year randomized trial of schoolMAX, the current study demonstrates the success of the three component implementation model in maintaining high levels of treatment fidelity by school staff across the school year. Implications for the use of this implementation model in enhancing execution of school-based interventions are discussed.

As the prevalence of autism spectrum disorder (ASD) continues to increase (Centers for Disease Control and Prevention, 2014), educators are faced with a growing challenge to meet and address the needs of children with ASD in public schools (White, Scahill, Klin, Koenig, & Volkmar, 2007). ASD is defined by core deficits in social interaction and communication and circumscribed behaviors and interests (APA, 2013). Children with high-

In: Autism Spectrum Disorders
Editor: Arlene Valdez

ISBN: 978-1-63482-547-4

Chapter 6

Achieving and Maintaining Intervention Fidelity Using a Three-Component Implementation Model in a Comprehensive School-Based Psychosocial Treatment for Children with High-Functioning ASD

Marcus L. Thomeer[1*], *Jonathan D. Rodgers*[1], *Christopher Lopata*[1], *Andrew T. Nelson*[2] *and Adam J. Booth*[2]
[1]Institute for Autism Research, Canisius College, Buffalo, NY, US
[2]University at Buffalo, State University of New York, Buffalo, NY, US

* Corresponding Author: M. Thomeer, thomeerm@canisius.edu.

functioning autism spectrum disorder (HFASD) present a unique dilemma for educators. They have average to above average language and cognitive skills (Klin, McPartland, & Volkmar, 2005) but may not reach their expected academic potential (Estes, Rivera, Bryan, Cali, & Dawson, 2011) due to their inability to navigate and interact appropriately in the classroom environment (Marans, Rubin, & Laurent, 2005). Examples of social deficits that negatively impact their school functioning include impaired turn-taking, listening, cooperating, and transitioning (Ostmeyer & Scarpa, 2012), poor nonverbal communication (Lindner & Rosen, 2006), and the tendency to focus intensely on a limited range of topics (South, Ozonoff, & McMahon, 2005).

In order for children with HFASD to be successful both academically and socially, school professionals must develop and implement programming that addresses their social deficits. Unfortunately, White, Scahill, and colleagues (2007) found that even though more children with HFASD are being identified to receive special education services, most are not receiving the adequate amount of services necessary to address their social communication and interaction deficits. Recent federal mandates, such as No Child Left Behind (2002) and The Individuals with Disabilities Education Act (IDEA, 2004), require the implementation of evidenced-based practices in schools for children classified with a disability thereby placing more onus on teachers to address the needs of children with HFASD. A body of research demonstrating effective strategies (e.g.,, explicit instruction, modeling, role-playing, repeated practice) exists to remediate social deficits of children with HFASD (see Lopata, Volker, Toomey, Chow, & Thomeer, 2008; Odom, Collet-Klingenberg, Rogers, & Hatton, 2010; Rao, Beidel, & Murray, 2008; Reichow & Volkmar, 2010). However, the translation of these strategies into established and validated protocols for implementation in school settings is in its infancy and has shown mixed results (Bellini, Peters, Benner, & Hopf, 2007; Reichow & Volkmar, 2010). Bellini et al. (2007) suggested that a majority of interventions have been unsuccessful due to the lack of intervention intensity, poor treatment adherence, and failure to integrate the intervention across the school day. Reichow and Volkmar (2010) identified social skills groups as an evidence-based practice in their review yet stressed the difficulty in replicating research validated in the lab or clinic into authentic environments where the school staff have many responsibilities beyond the intervention. For teacher implemented social skill interventions to be successful, the feasibility and social validity of these interventions in school settings must be established (Lang et al., 2010; Reichow & Volkmar, 2010). In a review of teacher involvement in 49 studies involving teachers of children with ASD, Lang and colleagues (2010) found that it was not enough to provide evidenced-based practices for schools if the school staff are not trained and supported in their implementation.

For schools to effectively implement evidenced-based strategies, Kasari and Smith (2013) stress the need for researchers and educational professionals to develop interventions collaboratively. Interventions must go beyond social skill instruction and create opportunities within the school day for children with HFASD to practice and transfer taught skills across multiple contexts (Bellini et al., 2007; Hart & Whalon, 2011; Thomeer, 2012). While procedures and dosage for implementing the core components of the intervention should be clearly specified and manualized (Durlak & DuPre, 2008; Kasari & Smith, 2013), some flexibility should be allowed in the logistical aspects of the intervention (i.e., who, when, and where to conduct core elements of the intervention; Kasari & Smith, 2013; Ringwalt et al., 2003).

Program Development

Schools provide an environment rich with opportunities for social interaction and populated by professionals and para-professionals with basic training, experience, and an interest in helping children (Kasari & Smith, 2013). Children also spend a majority of their time in schools (at least 9-10 months a year). In light of this, schools are an ideal setting for interventions. Odom, Boyd, Hall, and Hume (2010) recommend that interventions for children with ASD be comprehensive and address core ASD features and broader learning/development. These comprehensive treatments are comprised of multiple intervention components that target multiple domains and are typically applied intensively for an extended period of time (Odom, Boyd et al., 2010; Smith et al., 2007). Additionally, these treatments have a specified framework and manual, operationalized content and implementation procedures, and a method of assessing treatment fidelity via formalized measures (Odom, Boyd et al., 2010).

In identifying treatment components to be used for children with HFASD, Lopata and colleagues (2008) recommend that school-based interventions be adapted from university-clinic based interventions empirically validated through clinical trials (e.g.,, Frankel et al., 2010; Koenig et al., 2010; Lopata et al., 2010; Thomeer, Lopata et al., 2012). Validated interventions include high levels of structure, direct instruction, modeling, role-playing, repeated practice, reinforcement, and parent training/involvement (Reichow, Steiner, &

Volkmar, 2013; White, Koenig, & Scahill, 2007). A key issue in developing and implementing comprehensive school-based intervention components is to actively engage school staff and seek their input as to how to implement the programs while balancing academic needs and mandates (Lopata, Thomeer, Volker, Lee, Smith et al., 2013; Lopata et al., 2012; Thomeer, 2012).

Program Implementation

For an intervention to be maximally successful, researchers suggest that implementation procedures matter (Durlak & DuPre, 2008). Common elements of implementation identified include (1) instruction in intervention procedures; (2) monitoring of intervention fidelity, and (3) ongoing consultation and technical support (Bryson et al., 2007; Durlak & DuPre, 2008; Lopata et al., 2008).

Instruction

School staff will need support in the form of training if they are to be successful in implementing interventions (Durlak & DuPre, 2008; Kasari & Smith, 2013). Unfortunately, details of effective training components are infrequently reported (Lang et al., 2010). Fixsen, Naoom, Blase, Friedman, and Wallace (2005) emphasize techniques such as modeling, role-playing and performance feedback to help providers master the specific intervention skills. Lopata and colleagues have integrated these techniques and demonstrated that didactic instruction, observation of the implementation of treatment components, practicing components and establishing provider proficiency were effective in yielding high levels of treatment fidelity as well as significant treatment gains for children with HFASD as part of a summer treatment program (see review Lopata, Thomeer, Volker, & Lee, 2013). These techniques were also effective at producing high levels of fidelity in a comprehensive school-based intervention (Lopata, Thomeer, Volker, Lee, Smith et al., 2013; Lopata et al., 2012).

Treatment Fidelity

Durlak and DuPre (2008) conducted a large meta-analysis of the link between psychosocial outcomes and intervention fidelity. They found a very strong relationship between intervention outcomes and intervention fidelity across a wide variety of programs. Specifically, programs with high intervention fidelity demonstrated two-to-three times the effectiveness compared to programs that did not reliably or systematically assess treatment fidelity. Within research in ASD, there has been an increased awareness of the importance in evaluating and reporting treatment fidelity (Neely, Davis, Davis, & Rispoli, 2015). Reichow (2011) sets the benchmark to demonstrate adequate intervention fidelity at greater than .80. To ensure treatment implementation is consistent throughout the intervention, Durlak and DuPre (2008) and Fixsen et al. (2005) recommend that fidelity data be collected at multiple time points thereby allowing supervisors to evaluate and respond to variability.

Consultation and Support

A meta-analysis by Solomon, Klein, and Politylo (2012), has demonstrated that performance feedback given throughout a classroom intervention is effective at increasing and maintaining treatment fidelity. Dufrene, Lestremau, and Zoder-Martell (2014) found direct instruction, performance feedback, and modeling were critical to effective usage of new procedures by classroom teachers. In addition, consultation should provide ongoing opportunities to problem solve children's response to the intervention and to modify intervention targets and goals based on the child's progress (Lopata et al., 2008). The consistent and ongoing communication with the facilitators, according to Fixsen et al. (2005), is critical for maintaining their engagement in the intervention.

Educator-Mediated Intervention Studies

There has been limited research on comprehensive educator-mediated treatment interventions for children with HFASD. In a series of studies, Lopata, Thomeer, Volker, Lee, Smith and colleagues (2012, 2013) describe the feasibility and initial efficacy of a comprehensive school-based psychosocial intervention (schoolMAX) that was systematically developed in collaboration with education personnel (see Thomeer, 2012) and implemented across a 10-month school year. The schoolMAX program includes five active educator-implemented treatment components (i.e., social skills groups, therapeutic activities, individual daily notes, face and voice emotion recognition instruction, and parent training). These components address core and associated features of children with HFASDs. Results from these two studies indicated high treatment acceptability (school staff, parents and children reported high satisfaction with the schoolMAX protocol and implementation) and feasibility (high levels of treatment fidelity and teacher- and parent-reported acceptability and satisfaction). Preliminary analysis of the children's exposure to schoolMAX revealed gains in identification of targeted social skills, face-emotion recognition accuracy, and teacher and parent-reported social behaviors, as well as reductions in ASD-associated features.

Laugeson, Ellingsen, Sanderson, Tucci, and Bates (2014) modified their *Program for the Education and Enrichment of Relational Skills* (*PEERS®*) for implementation in a school setting. Social skills instruction was provided by classroom teachers and instructional aides for 30-minutes daily, including modeling, role-plays by the teachers, and performance feedback to students. Forty adolescents with HFASD were the primary participants. Rehearsal activities were also included though the duration and content of these activities was not described. The students were given socialization homework related to the social skill being targeted and parents were provided information on the weekly topic. Parent, teacher, and self-reports were compared to an active treatment group of 33 adolescents with HFASD receiving an alternative treatment (*Super Skills*; Coucouvanis, 2005). Results indicated significant gains in social functioning on a variety of measures for the modified *PEERS®* program. The school staff providing the intervention were given initial instruction in the intervention and then weekly supervision with the research supervisor who was a co-developer of the program. Treatment fidelity was monitored to ensure major instructional components were covered during lessons.

These studies highlight the potential for educator-mediated programs and the need for disseminating detailed procedures regarding the level of implementation monitoring and support required to maximize outcomes. The current chapter will describe the elements and implementation of a comprehensive school-based intervention (schoolMAX) and its three component implementation model. The implementation model consists of 1) instruction, observation, planning, and practice; 2) treatment fidelity monitoring; and 3) consultative feedback. Data from the first year of a randomized controlled trial (RCT) into the program's efficacy will be used to demonstrate how this model resulted in high levels of treatment fidelity across the intervention.

Description of schoolMAX

The schoolMAX program (Lopata, Thomeer, Volker, Lee, Smith et al., 2013; Lopata et al., 2012; Thomeer, 2012) is a manualized comprehensive school-based intervention conducted across a 10-month school year. It is specifically designed to target the core and associated features of children with HFASD via five active treatment components: (1) social skills groups; (2) face-voice emotion recognition instruction; (3) therapeutic activities; (4) individualized daily notes; and (5) parent training. The schoolMAX manual delineates the standardized content, instructional procedures, and the frequency and duration for implementing each of these five components. In addition to the standardized protocol, the manual allows the flexibility to identify which staff implements the component and when and where it will be conducted. Descriptions of each of the five active schoolMAX treatment components, who typically leads each component, and their dosage parameters are as follows.

Social Skills Groups (SSGs)

SSGs are conducted three times per week for a total of 60-90 minutes with no more than 6 students and are led by a related services professional (e.g.,, school psychologist, speech/language pathologist, school counselor, or social worker) and may be assisted by a paraprofessional (e.g.,, teacher assistant, teacher aide). The content of each SSG is derived from *Skillstreaming* (Goldstein, McGinnis, Sprafkin, Gershaw, & Klein, 1997), a structured curriculum that uses teaching, modeling, role-playing, performance feedback, and transfer of learning to improve the interpersonal skills of children (McGinnis & Goldstein, 1997). Each SSG begins with a review of rules (e.g.,, be actively involved, stay in seat/area) and then follows the nine steps of the *Skillstreaming* instructional protocol (Goldstein et al., 1997). The nine steps are: (1) define the skill; (2) model the skill; (3) establish trainee skill need; (4) select role-player; (5) set up the role-play; (6) conduct the role-play; (7) provide performance feedback; (8) assign skill homework; and (9) select next role-player. A total of 26 social skills from *Skillstreaming* are targeted (beginning with basic to more complex skills) across the school year. Each social skill aligns with specific diagnostic and associated features of children with HFASD (Lopata, Thomeer, Volker, & Lee, 2013). The last two-to-three minutes of each session include a short debrief during which the SSG leader reviews the group's performance and discusses how participants can use the skill taught that day across the school day.

Face and Voice Emotion Recognition Instruction (*Mind Reading*; *MR*)

MR is an interactive software program designed to teach recognition of a broad range of basic and complex emotions in facial and vocal formats (Baron-Cohen, Golan, Wheelwright, & Hill, 2004). Students receive *MR* instruction individually via a computer for two to three sessions a week for a total of 60 minutes per week. Each session has specific tasks and/or lessons that have to be completed and each student's completion of the designated session tasks are monitored by a school team member (e.g.,, paraprofessional). Students earn tokens for correctly answering questions in *MR* program lessons and quizzes. Over the course of the school year, students are specifically taught 100 *MR* emotions.

Therapeutic Activities (TAs)

TAs are cooperative group activities specifically designed for the students to practice and reinforce skills taught during the SSGs. TAs are conducted twice per week for a total of 40-60 minutes and are led by a designated school team member. TAs require at least two students but can be conducted with an entire special education or general education class. Each TA lesson plan describes the activity, its purpose, skill targeted, materials needed, deficit addressed, and procedures for conducting the activity. For each TA, the facilitator reviews the activity rules, content, and purpose, and then discusses with the target student(s) how she/he could use taught skills during the activity. The designated facilitator(s) must maintain close proximity to the target student(s) to ensure they are able to provide reinforcement and corrective feedback for any exhibition of target skills. The last two-to-three minutes of the TA involves a debriefing on how the TA went and how students could use the target skills across the school day.

Individual Daily Note (IDN)

The IDN is a behavioral reinforcement system implemented to increase the student's use and practice of taught skills and reduce her/his challenging behaviors. The IDN is implemented across the school day by all members of the student's educational team; however, the student's primary teacher takes the lead role in determining and monitoring progress on targets. Each IDN is individualized to the unique needs of the specific student with HFASD and consists of three-to-five operationally-defined targets. At least two of the IDN targets must address social behaviors (e.g.,, having a conversation or looking at person who is talking). Additional targets address child-specific problematic behaviors (e.g.,, organization, following directions, or completing work). The IDN divides each student's school day into intervals and the students are monitored and given feedback by school staff during each interval for their adherence to IDN target criteria. If the child meets at least 75% of her/his targets for the day then the student is reinforced at home for her/his school-based performance on the IDN.

Parent Training (PT)

PT group sessions seek to inform parents of procedures and content of schoolMAX and to increase parental knowledge of strategies to help their child with HFASD improve his/her social and behavioral performance at home and school. Ten 60 minute PT sessions are conducted monthly across the school year and are led by at least one member of a school's educational team. PT content and instructional procedures are manualized to ensure delivery of consistent content by all participating school teams. In each session, the facilitator provides a brief discussion on schoolMAX progress and session agenda, presents and discusses lesson content, leads parents into creating a plan to integrate session content into their daily routines, and reviews each parent's implementation plans of session content.

(For a further description of the schoolMAX program and documentation of its feasibility and initial efficacy see Lopata, Thomeer, Volker, Lee, Smith et al., 2013; Lopata et al., 2012; Thomeer, 2012).

hools total; four schools in one district and two in the other). Children were cruited by having the director of special education in targeted districts send 1 invitation letter to parents of children receiving special education services. arents then contacted the researchers and were given information about the udy (purpose, inclusion criteria, procedures, etc.). Interested parents then ubmitted documentation of a prior clinical diagnosis of ASD, sychoeducational evaluations, and a background form. Senior research team nembers then reviewed documentation for likelihood of a child's qualification or the study and likely candidates were invited to complete a formal ssessment (cognitive, language, and ASD diagnostic). Inclusion criteria were Wechsler Intelligence Scales for Children - Fourth Edition (Wechsler, 2003) short-form full scale IQ > 70, Perceptual Reasoning or Verbal Comprehension Index $\geq$ 80; Comprehensive Assessment of Spoken Language (Carrow-Woolfolk, 1999) short-form Receptive or Expressive language composite > 75; and scores meeting ASD criteria on the Autism Diagnostic Interview-Revised (Rutter, LeCouteur, & Lord, 2003).

School buildings were randomly assigned to either the schoolMAX program or a control (*business as usual*) condition. Three schools were assigned to schoolMAX and three to control. Thirteen children (11 boys and 2 girls) were in school buildings conducting schoolMAX. Two of the schools (school #1 and school #3) had five children each, while one of the schools (school #2) had three children. Approximately three school professionals were identified per child to facilitate schoolMAX. See Table 1 for a breakdown of participating school staff characteristics. In general, school staff were similar across the three schools. School staff averaged 16.6 years of education and 13.1 years of experience. Participating staff ranged widely in the amount of training they received working with children with HFASD prior to schoolMAX, such that approximately a third reported less than 5 hours, a third reported between 5 and 20 hours, and a third reported over 20 hours. Across all three schools, participating staff included teachers, paraprofessionals, speech and language professionals, school psychologists, social workers, and special education teachers.

Implementation

In all three schools, implementation of schoolMAX followed the model described above. No modifications were made to the implementation model or schoolMAX program.

schoolMAX Implementation Model

The schoolMAX implementation protocol consists of a three component process that includes 1) instruction, observation, planning, and practice; 2) treatment fidelity monitoring; and 3) consultative feedback. Instruction, observation, practice, and planning are used to build school staff knowledge and proficiency and adapt the intervention to the participating school environment (flexibility). Treatment fidelity is monitored throughout implementation by research clinicians to ensure the intervention protocol is conducted consistently and reliably. These research clinicians monitor fidelity while also providing ongoing modeling and support. Third, regular consultative feedback on provider proficiency is delivered to school staff by the senior research team. This feedback reviews ongoing intervention fidelity, problem-solves implementation issues, and evaluates student progress.

Instruction, Observation, Planning, and Practice

In the summer months prior to implementing schoolMAX, all participating school staff receive 30 hours of training. The first ten hours cover: (1) diagnostic characteristics and features of ASD; (2) research on social skill interventions for children with HFASD; (3) development and previous implementation of the schoolMAX program; and (4) specific implementation instruction in the schoolMAX treatment components. Implementation instruction includes manualized procedures for implementing the components, documenting treatment component dosage, and procedures used to monitor treatment fidelity. Next, educational team members observe live and video examples of the schoolMAX components being implemented.

After completing observations, meetings are held with the school staff from each school to determine who the school facilitators will be for each treatment component, the times and space to be used, the resources needed, times and location for the future consultation meetings, and a dissemination plan to inform the general school staff about schoolMAX and what it entails for the school community. In identifying facilitators, SSGs are generally conducted by related-service providers (speech-language pathologist or school psychologist), *MR* is implemented by classroom aides, TAs are conducted by teachers (general and special education) in collaboration with related-service providers (social worker, intervention/consultant teachers), the IDN is implemented, managed, and coordinated by the student's primary classroom teacher, and PT is co-facilitated by related-service providers (speech-language pathologist, school psychologist, or social worker) and a member of the research team.

It is in these planning sessions that flexibility in component configuration is decided. For example, in identifying facilitators for the SSGs, the school psychologist may have limited time to run social skill groups twice a week so may split leading the social skill group sessions with the school's social worker. For the IDN, while the teacher may be the point person, a paraprofessional in the classroom may assist in implementation and monitoring. In identifying schedules for implementation, while *MR* is to be conducted each week for 60 minutes total, it can be conducted in three 20 minute sessions each week or two 30 minute sessions each week. This flexibility ensures that the manualized procedures can be integrated into the child's daily schedule by various members of the child's educational team. Once schedules and facilitators are determined, materials for implementing components (i.e., SSG social skills lists and posters, group rule posters, laptops to conduct *MR* sessions, parent training slides and DVD) are distributed.

Once facilitators are designated, they practice their component while research staff monitor their proficiency of implementation. Research staff use standardized fidelity sheets developed for each treatment component. Two to three research assistants serve as "children" in these practice sessions. All school facilitators have to score at least 90% on these fidelity observations before they are considered sufficiently competent to implement the component. During training, facilitators must continue to conduct practice sessions until they achieve 90%. Between these sessions, senior research team give performance feedback and model any specific elements missed.

Treatment Fidelity Monitoring

Research assistants monitor school staff adherence to the schoolMAX protocol using standardized fidelity sheets. Research assistants are trained to meet the same intervention proficiency as the school staff. The fidelity sheets document the specific steps and sequence for each component in the manualized protocol. For example, the SSG fidelity sheet lists the step-by-step procedures required to conduct the group. This includes reviewing the rules for the group, conducting the nine *Skillstreaming* steps, and leading the group wrap-up discussion. Fidelity is scored using a percentage of procedural elements completed correctly by the facilitator. Across the schoolMAX

program, treatment fidelity is assessed once per three SSGs and *M*. and three times per eight TAs. IDN fidelity is assessed for two hours per child. For PT sessions, fidelity is monitored in five of the ten ses school. In order to confirm inter-observer agreement, 20% of treatme observations are completed by two independent research simultaneously.

Consultative Feedback

Throughout the school year, all facilitators participate in bi- consultation meetings that are led by each student's primary classroom and a senior research team member. Consultative feedback generall from 30-45 minutes depending on the degree of feedback nec Treatment fidelity data are presented and direct performance feedba specific program implementation is given. These consultation meeting provide the opportunity to review child individual behavioral progress from the IDN and problem solve any issues related to participants. IDN adjusted based on behavioral progress (e.g.,, a behavioral target with performance may be modified by reducing the number of prompts, incre the length of the interval, or replacing the target). The first two consult meetings focus on determining initial IDN targets, intervals for monitorin child's behavior, and baseline criteria for each target.

Consultative feedback, in addition to the bi-weekly meetings, includes direct support during intervention component delivery. Se research team members attend intervention elements and provide immed performance feedback to facilitators. Research assistants model parts of intervention where necessary at the discretion of the senior research team the facilitators.

Data Illustration

Participants and Inclusion Criteria

The implementation data from the first year of a four-year RCT of th schoolMAX program are used to illustrate the potential efficacy of th described model. Twenty elementary school children (18 boys and 2 girls ages 7-12) with HFASD were recruited from two public school districts (si

Facilitator Training Proficiency

All school facilitators' initial implementation proficiency met or exceeded the required 90% threshold. The first data point in each of the Figures (1-4) represents the average initial proficiency during training of the primary facilitators for each element.

Table 1. Participating School Staff Characteristics

Characteristic	Overall	School #1	School #2	School #3
Number of staff involved in schoolMAX	37	13	11	13
Staff years of education	16.6 (2.4)	16.9 (1.9)	16.1 (2.9)	16.8 (2.4)
Years of experience	13.1 (6.5)	10.9 (5.4)	16.5 (7.6)	12.5 (5.7)
Previous training with ASD (# of hours)				
<5 =	12	7	3	2
5-10 =	7	0	4	3
10-20 =	8	3	0	5
20-30 =	3	1	1	1
30-40 =	0	0	0	0
>40 =	7	2	3	2
Position at school				
Classroom Teacher	12	5	3	4
Paraprofessional	12	3	5	4
Reading Specialist	2	1	0	1
School Psychologist	2	0	1	1
School Social Worker	2	1	0	1
Special Education Teacher	3	1	1	1
Speech/Language Professional	4	2	1	1

Treatment Fidelity

Figures 1-4 illustrate trends in the average monthly percentage of treatment fidelity for four of the treatment components (SSG, TA, MR and IDN) in each school. Because PT occurred less frequently and was monitored and co-facilitated by research staff, it is reported separately. Twenty percent of all treatment fidelity observations were conducted by two independent research assistants. Average inter-observer agreement exceeded 90% for all elements.

SSGs Fidelity

Average overall SSG fidelity was 88% across the school-based intervention. School #1 averaged 90%, school #2 averaged 83%, and school #3 averaged 90%. Monthly percentages are graphed in Figure 1. Month-to-month average SSG treatment fidelity exceeded 85% in school #1 and school #3. School #2 had two consecutive months (month #3 and #4) where average fidelity dropped below 80%. Immediate performance feedback along with additional support and modeling was provided; following this, fidelity in month #5 exceeded 80% and months #6-#9 exceeded 90%.

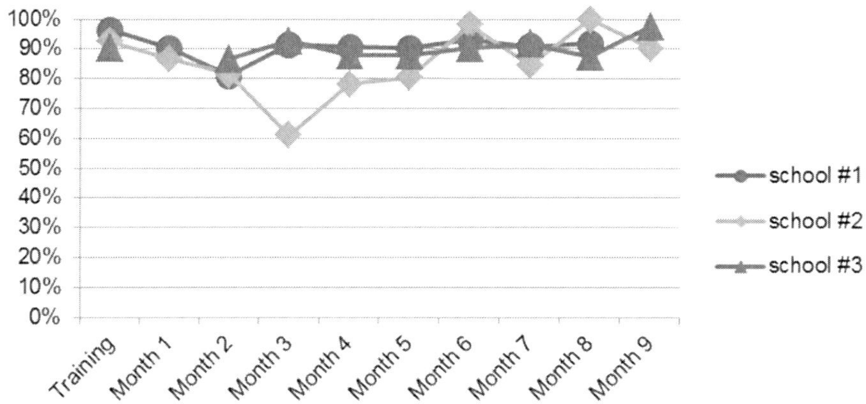

Figure 1. Social skills group (SSG) month-to-month treatment fidelity.

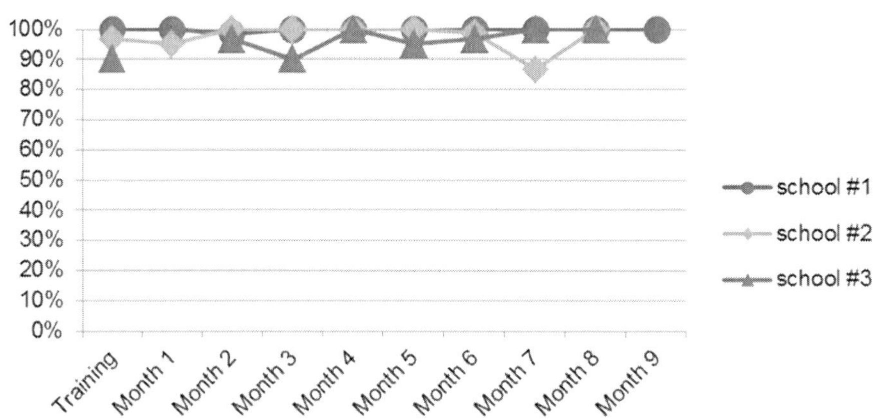

Figure 2. Therapeutic activity (TA) month-to-month treatment fidelity.

TA Fidelity

Average overall TA fidelity was 99% across the school-based intervention. Of the three schools: school #1 averaged 100%, school #2 averaged 98%, and school #3 averaged 99% across the school year. The monthly percentages are graphed in Figure 2. Month-to-month average TA treatment fidelity exceeded 85% in all schools.

MR Fidelity

Average overall *MR* fidelity was 98% across the school-based intervention. Of the three schools: school #1 averaged 99%, school #2 averaged 98%, and school #3 averaged 97% across the school year. The monthly percentages are graphed in Figure 3. Month-to-month average *MR* treatment fidelity exceeded 85% in all schools.

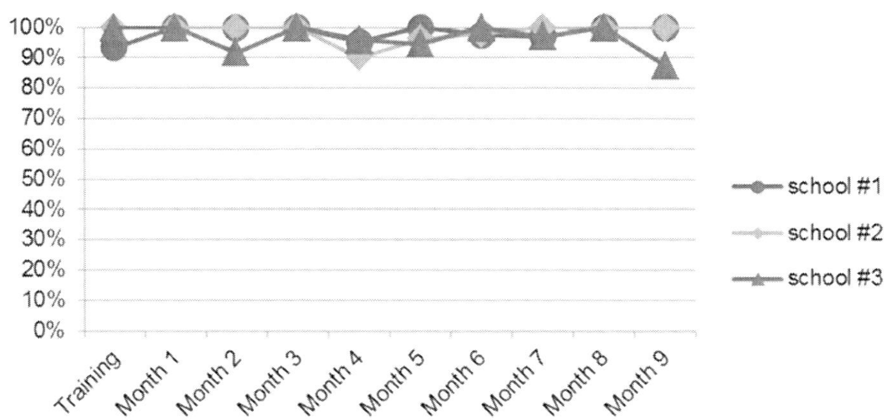

Figure 3. *Mind Reading (MR)* month-to-month treatment fidelity.

IDN Fidelity

Average overall IDN fidelity was 95% across the school-based intervention. Of the three schools: school #1 averaged 96%, school #2 averaged 97%, and school #3 averaged 93% across the school year. The monthly percentages are graphed in Figure 4. Month-to-month average IDN treatment fidelity exceeded 85% in all schools.

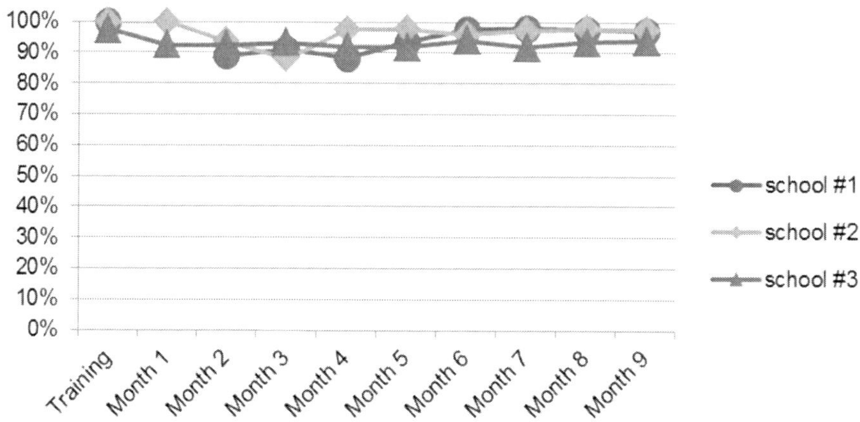

Figure 4. Individualized daily note (IDN) month-to-month treatment fidelity.

PT Fidelity

Average overall PT fidelity was 94% across the school-based intervention. Of the three schools: school #1 and #3 (who ran joint PT sessions) had a combined average of 98% and school #2 averaged 91%. Of the ten PT fidelity observations only one observation, in school #2, was below 85% (during month 3 of the intervention). The facilitator from school #2 was given performance feedback and fidelity exceeded 85% in all subsequent observations.

Summary

The data illustrates the success of the implementation model in establishing and maintaining high intervention fidelity for the schoolMAX program. Average treatment fidelity ranged from 88% to 100% across components. Month-to-month average treatment fidelity in SSG and PT briefly dropped below 85%, but was remediated with performance feedback. Overall results highlight the potential effectiveness of training and ongoing performance feedback on establishing and maintaining intervention fidelity.

Discussion and Recommendations

The current chapter describes a systematic training and implementation model for an educator-mediated comprehensive intervention for children with HFASD. It has described the schoolMAX program, discussed the three-part implementation model, and illustrated the potential effectiveness of this model with treatment fidelity data from the first year of a four-year RCT into the efficacy of schoolMAX. schoolMAX and the implementation model has been supported by two previous studies of its feasibility as a treatment for children with HFASD (see Lopata, Thomeer, Volker, Lee, Smith et al., 2013; Lopata et al., 2012). Average implementation fidelity was above recommended standards (Reichow, 2011) for all elements in those initial studies and continues to meet these standards in the first year of the current RCT. Specifically, in the current study, three of the five (MR, TA, and IDN) components averaged month-to-month treatment fidelity exceeding 85%. While two elements' (SSG and PT) average treatment fidelity fell below this criterion briefly, they returned to previously high levels with performance feedback and support. The schoolMAX implementation model provides a consistent opportunity for the senior research team to respond to drops in intervention fidelity during the bi-weekly meetings and ongoing consultation. As noted by Fixsen et al. (2005), school facilitators tend to respond positively when communication and performance feedback is ongoing and includes direct support.

The current chapter is the first detailed illustration of implementation procedures for an educator-mediated comprehensive intervention for children with HFASD. In general, limited research has been conducted on educator-mediated interventions with this population, and the description of training processes in the research available is sparse (Kasari & Smith, 2013). For example, Laugeson et al. (2014) describes an educator-mediated intervention, but the description of training procedures is limited to a brief mention of the duration of training and supervision. Given the critical influence of treatment fidelity on intervention efficacy (Durlak & DuPre, 2008), training procedures for intervention programs must be well-elucidated and replicable, particularly when interventions are conducted outside of a clinical-research environment (i.e., schools). While the space available in a peer-reviewed publication may not be sufficient to fully describe an implementation model, at minimum a supplemental appendix or enhanced methods sections should be provided with a full description for any potential school-based intervention for children with HFASD.

Limitations and Future Studies

The current description of the implementation model for schoolMAX is limited by the inclusion of only one year of example data. As the current model is being used in a four-year RCT, additional implementation information and outcome data will be presented in future publications. The present chapter uses initial implementation fidelity data to elucidate the possible success of the implementation model; however, there is no way to account for threats to internal/external validity in attributing intervention success to the implementation model, thus these data should be considered illustrative only. The final analysis of the schoolMAX RCT results should consider treatment fidelity as a potential covariate of overall efficacy as suggested by Durlak and DuPre (2008). Additionally, the psychometric characteristics of the fidelity measures used in this implementation model should be evaluated.

Upon validation of schoolMAX with the three component implementation model, a future study could compare conducting the program using all three implementation components to conducting the program using only one of the components (i.e., training, observation, planning, and practice). This could provide evidence for the necessity of the full implementation model. Subsequent studies could also explore the impact of prior teacher experience on the intensity required for the implementation components.

Enhancements to the Implementation Model

The current implementation model appears to be successful at establishing and maintaining a high level of treatment fidelity. The following additional enhancements may improve its effectiveness.

(1) *Performance criteria for retraining.* The current model relies on senior research team members' discretion to make decisions regarding provision of additional support and retraining. Setting performance criteria that trigger an automatic increase in support could make the model more viable for application with other interventions beyond schoolMAX. For example, a facilitator with a monthly or weekly fidelity average of less than 85% could automatically lead to additional support, modeling, and performance feedback from research staff.

(2) *Description of implementation model and performance feedback.* A potential enhancement to the implementation model would be to include as part of didactic instruction an exposition of how performance feedback is given. This would include a specific review of fidelity monitoring procedures, an example of performance feedback, and a description of support provided.

(3) *Establish revision criteria for the IDN.* A third possible enhancement to the current implementation model would be to develop a formalized process for revising IDN targets. While school facilitators and the senior research team review and make adjustments to IDN targets based on the data of student's performance in bi-weekly meetings, more formalized criteria as to when to make adjustments may be beneficial. For example, when a child achieves greater than 90% on a particular target over a set period of time, the team would know to review the target and make modifications. These criteria would not demand a modification be made, but would alert the senior research team and facilitators to review the individual's performance with that target.

Conclusion

The increase in the prevalence of children with HFASD is a critical concern for educators. The demonstration of feasibility and social validity of comprehensive interventions in school settings must be a priority if interventions are going to be validated and disseminated effectively (Reichow and Volkmar, 2010). The present chapter demonstrates how the three component implementation model is potentially effective in ensuring high treatment fidelity with educators executing a comprehensive school-based intervention. The schoolMAX three component implementation model incorporates ubiquitous elements of intervention training (i.e., initial training, planning, etc.), with increasingly reported elements (treatment fidelity monitoring), and direct consultation and feedback (consultative feedback). These three components are supported by a wide range of intervention implementation research (Durlak & DuPre, 2008; Kasari & Smith, 2013; Lang et al., 2010) and have been effective in eliciting positive treatment responses in past studies (Lopata, Thomeer, Volker, Lee, Smith et al., 2013; Lopata et al., 2012). The current chapter provides a framework for other interventions to use and future studies to expand and replicate.

Acknowledgments

The research reported in this chapter was supported by Department of Education, Institute of Education Sciences Grant R324A130216. Findings and conclusions are those of the authors and do not necessarily reflect the views of the funding agency. The authors declare no conflicts of interest.

References

American Psychiatric Association (2013). *Diagnostic and statistical manual of mental disorders* (5th ed.). Arlington, VA: American Psychiatric Association.

Baron-Cohen, S., Golan, O., Wheelwright, S., & Hill, J. J. (2004). *Mind reading: The interactive guide to emotions.* London, UK: Jessica Kingsley Publishing.

Bellini, S., Peters, J. K., Benner, L., & Hopf, A. (2007). A meta-analysis of school-based social skills interventions for children with autism spectrum disorders. *Remedial and Special Education, 28*(3), 153-162. doi: 10.1177/07419325070280030401.

Bryson, S. E., Koegel, L. K., Koegel, R. L., Openden, D., Smith, I. M., & Nefdt, N. (2007). Large scale dissemination and community implementation of pivotal response treatment: Program description and preliminary data. *Research and Practice for Persons with Severe Disabilities, 32*(2), 142-153.

Carrow-Woolfolk, E. (1999). *Comprehensive assessment of spoken language.* Circle Pines, MN: American Guidance Service.

Center for Disease Control and Prevention. (2014). Prevalence of autism spectrum disorders - autism and developmental disabilities monitoring network, 14 Sites, United States, 2010.

Coucouvanis, J. (2005). *Super Skills: A social skills group program for children with Asperger syndrome, high-functioning autism and related challenges.* Shawnee Mission: Autism Asperger Publishing Company.

Dufrene, B. A., Lestremau, L., & Zoder-Martell, K. (2014). Direct behavioral consultation: Effects on teachers' praise and student disruptive behavior. *Psychology in the Schools, 51*(6), 567-580. doi: 10.1002/pits.21768.

Durlak, J. A., & DuPre, E. P. (2008). Implementation matters: A review of research on the influence of implementation on program outcomes and the factors affecting implementation. *American Journal of Community Psychology, 41*(3-4), 327-350. doi: 10.1007/s10464-008-9165-0.

Estes, A., Rivera, V., Bryan, M., Cali, P., & Dawson, G. (2011). Discrepancies between academic achievement and intellectual ability in higher-functioning school-aged children with autism apectrum disorder. *Journal of Autism and Developmental Disorders, 41*(8), 1044-1052. doi: 10.1007/s10803-010-1127-3.

Fixsen, D. L., Naoom, S. F., Blase, K. A., Friedman, R. M., & Wallace, F. (2005). *Implementation research: A synthesis of the literature*. Tampa, FL: University of South Florida, Louis de la Parte Florida Mental Health Institute, The National Implementation Research Network (FMHI Publication #231): Retrieved from http://nirn.fmhi.usf.edu/resources/publications/Monograph/pdf/monograph_full.pdf.

Frankel, F., Myatt, R., Sugar, C., Whitham, C., Gorospe, C. M., & Laugeson, E. (2010). A randomized controlled study of parent-assisted Children's Friendship Training with children having autism spectrum disorders. *Journal of Autism and Developmental Disorders, 40*(7), 827-842. doi: 10.1007/s10803-009-0932-z.

Goldstein, A. P., McGinnis, E., Sprafkin, R. P., Gershaw, N. J., & Klein, P. (1997). *Skillstreaming the adolescent: New strategies and perspectives for teaching prosocial skills (Rev. ed.)*. Champaign, Il: Research Press.

Hart, J. E., & Whalon, K. J. (2011). Creating social opportunities for students with autism spectrum disorder in inclusive settings. *Intervention in School and Clinic, 46*(5), 273-279. doi: 10.1177/1053451210395382.

Individuals with Disabilities in Education Act of 2004, Pub. L. No.108-446, § 101, 118 Stat. 2647 C.F.R. (2004).

Kasari, C., & Smith, T. (2013). Interventions in schools for children with autism spectrum disorder: Methods and recommendations. *Autism, 17*(3), 254-267. doi: 10.1177/1362361312470496.

Klin, A., McPartland, J., & Volkmar, F. (2005). Asperger syndrome. In F. R. Volkmar, R. Paul, A. Klin & D. Cohen (Eds.), *Handbook of autism and pervasive developmental disorders: Vol 1. Diagnosis, development, neurobiology, and behavior* (3rd ed., Vol. 1, pp. 88-125). Hoboken, NJ: John Wiley & Sons.

Koenig, K., White, S. W., Pachler, M., Lau, M., Lewis, M., Klin, A., & Scahill, L. (2010). Promoting social skill development in children with pervasive developmental disorders: A feasibility and efficacy study. *Journal of Autism and Developmental Disorders, 40*(10), 1209-1218. doi: 10.1007/s10803-010-0979-x.

Lang, R., O'Reilly, M. F., Sigafoos, J., Machalicek, W., Rispoli, M., Shogren, K., Chan, J. M., Davis, T., Lancioni, G., & Hopkins, S. (2010). Review of teacher involvement in the applied intervention research for children with autism spectrum disorders. *Education and Training in Autism and Developmental Disabilities, 45*(2), 268-283.

Laugeson, E. A., Ellingsen, R., Sanderson, J., Tucci, L., & Bates, S. (2014). The ABC's of Teaching social skills to adolescents with autism spectrum disorder in the classroom: The UCLA PEERS® Program. *Journal of Autism and Developmental Disorders, 44*(9), 2244-2256. doi: 10.1007/s10803-014-2108-8.

Lindner, J. L., & Rosen, L. A. (2006). Decoding of emotion through facial expression, prosody and verbal content in children and adolescents with Asperger's syndrome. *Journal of Autism and Developmental Disorders, 36*(6), 769-777. doi: 10.1007/s10803-006-0105-2.

Lopata, C., Thomeer, M. L., Volker, M. A., & Lee, G. K. (2013). A manualized summer program for social skills in children with high-functioning ASD. In A. Scarpa, S. W. White & T. Attwood (Eds.), *CBT for children and adolescents with high-functioning autism spectrum disorders* (pp. 199-225). New York, NY: Guilford.

Lopata, C., Thomeer, M. L., Volker, M. A., Lee, G. K., Smith, T. H., Rodgers, J. D., Smith, R. A., Gullo, G., McDonald, C. A., Mirwis, J., & Toomey, J. A. (2013). Open-trial pilot study of a comprehensive school-based intervention for high-functioning autism spectrum disorders. *Remedial and Special Education, 34*(5), 269-281. doi: 10.1177/0741932512450518.

Lopata, C., Thomeer, M. L., Volker, M. A., Lee, G. K., Smith, T. H., Smith, R. A., McDonald, C. A., Rodgers, J. D., Lipinski, A. M., & Toomey, J. A. (2012). Feasibility and initial efficacy of a comprehensive school-based intervention for high-functioning autism spectrum disorders. *Psychology in the Schools, 49*(10), 963-974. doi: 10.1002/pits.21649.

Lopata, C., Thomeer, M. L., Volker, M. A., Toomey, J. A., Nida, R. E., Lee, G. K., Smerbeck, A. M., & Rodgers, J. D. (2010). RCT of a manualized social treatment for high-functioning autism spectrum disorders. *Journal of Autism and Developmental Disorders, 40*(11), 1297-1310. doi: 10.1007/s10803-010-0989-8.

Lopata, C., Volker, M. A., Toomey, J. A., Chow, S. Y., & Thomeer, M. L. (2008). Asperger's and other high functioning autism spectrum disorders: A review of group-based social enhancement research and a model for school-based social intervention. In D. H. Molina (Ed.), *School psychology: 21st century issues and challenges* (pp. 299-325). Hauppauge, NY: Nova Science.

Marans, W., Rubin, E., & Laurent, A. (2005). Addressing the social communication skills in individuals with high-functioning autism and Asperger syndrome: Critical priotities in educational programming. In F. R. Volkmar, R. Paul, A. Klin & D. Cohen (Eds.), *Handbook of autism and pervasive developmental disorders: Vol 2. Assessment, interventions, and policy* (3rd ed., Vol. 2, pp. 977-1002). Hoboken, NJ: John Wiley & Sons.

McGinnis, E., & Goldstein, A. P. (1997). *Skillstreaming the elementary school child: New strategies and perspectives for teaching prosocial skills (Rev. ed.)* Champaign, Il: Research Press.

Neely, L., Davis, H., Davis, J., & Rispoli, M. (2015). Review of reliability and treatment integrity trends in autism-focused research. *Research in Autism Spectrum Disorders, 9*, 1-12. doi: 10.1016/j.rasd.2014.09.011.

No Child Left Behind (NCLB) Act of 2001, Pub. L. No. 107-110, § 115, Stat. 1425 (2002).

Odom, S. L., Boyd, B. A., Hall, L. J., & Hume, K. (2010). Evaluation of comprehensive treatment models for individuals with autism spectrum disorders. *Journal of Autism and Developmental Disorders, 40*(4), 425-436. doi: 10.1007/s10803-009-0825-1.

Odom, S. L., Collet-Klingenberg, L., Rogers, S. J., & Hatton, D. D. (2010). Evidence-based practices in interventions for children and youth with autism spectrum disorders. *Preventing School Failure, 54*(4), 275-282. doi: 10.1080/10459881003785506.

Ostmeyer, K., & Scarpa, A. (2012). Examining school-based social skills program needs and barriers for students with high-functioning autism spectrum disorders using participatory action research. *Psychology in the Schools, 49*(10), 932-941. doi: 10.1002/pits.21646.

Rao, P. A., Beidel, D. C., & Murray, M. J. (2008). Social skills interventions for children with Asperger's syndrome or high-functioning autism: A review and recommendations. *Journal of Autism and Developmental Disorders, 38*(2), 353-361. doi: 10.1007/s10803-007-0402-4.

Reichow, B. (2011). Development, procedures, and application of the evaluative method for determining evidence-based practices in autism. In B. Reichow, P. Doehring, D. V. Cicchetti & F. R. Volkmar (Eds.), *Evidence-based practices and treatments for children with autism* (pp. 25-39). New York: Springer.

Reichow, B., Steiner, A. M., & Volkmar, F. (2013). Cochrane review: Social skills groups for people aged 6 to 21 with autism spectrum disorders

(ASD). *Evidence-Based Child Health: A Cochrane Review Journal, 8*(2), 266-315. doi: 10.1002/ebch.1903.

Reichow, B., & Volkmar, F. R. (2010). Social skills interventions for individuals with autism: Evaluation for evidence-based practices within a best evidence synthesis framework. *Journal of Autism and Developmental Disorders, 40*(2), 149-166. doi: 10.1007/s10803-009-0842-0.

Ringwalt, C. L., Ennett, S., Johnson, R., Rohrbach, L. A., Simons-Rudolph, A., Vincus, A., & Thorne, J. (2003). Factors associated with fidelity to substance use prevention curriculum guides in the nation's middle schools. *Health Education & Behavior, 30*(3), 375-391. doi: 10.1177/1090198103253627.

Rutter, M., LeCouteur, A., & Lord, C. (2003). *Autism Diagnostic Interview-Revised*. Los Angeles: Western Psychological Services.

Smith, T., Scahill, L., Dawson, G., Guthrie, D., Lord, C., Odom, S., Rogers, S., & Wagner, A. (2007). Designing research studies on psychosocial interventions in autism. *Journal of Autism and Developmental Disorders, 37*(2), 354-366. doi: 10.1007/s10803-006-0173-3.

Solomon, B. G., Klein, S. A., & Politylo, B. C. (2012). The effect of performance feedback on teachers' treatment integrity: A meta-analysis of the single-case literature. *School Psychology Review, 41*(2), 160-175.

South, M., Ozonoff, S., & McMahon, W. M. (2005). Repetitive behavior profiles in Asperger syndrome and high-functioning autism. *Journal of Autism and Developmental Disorders, 35*(2), 145-158. doi: 10.1007/s10803-005-1992-3.

Thomeer, M. L. (2012). Collaborative development and component trials of a comprehensive school-based intervention for children with HFASDs. *Psychology in the Schools, 49*(10), 955-962. doi: 10.1002/pits.21648

Thomeer, M. L., Lopata, C., Volker, M. A., Toomey, J. A., Lee, G. K., Smerbeck, A. M., Rodgers, J. D., McDonald, C. A., & Smith, R. A. (2012). Randomized clinical trial replication of a psychosocial treatment for children with high-functioning autism spectrum disorders. *Psychology in the Schools, 49*(10), 942-954. doi: 10.1002/pits.21647

Wechsler, D. (2003). *Wechsler Intelligence Scale for Children (4th ed.)*. San Antonio, TX: The Psychological Corporation.

White, S. W., Koenig, K., & Scahill, L. (2007). Social skills development in children with autism spectrum disorders: A review of the intervention research. *Journal of Autism and Developmental Disorders, 37*(10), 1858-1868. doi: 10.1007/s10803-006-0320-x

White, S. W., Scahill, L., Klin, A., Koenig, K., & Volkmar, F. R. (2007). Educational placements and service use patterns of individuals with autism spectrum disorders. *Journal of Autism and Developmental Disorders, 37*(8), 1403-1412. doi: 10.1007/s10803-006-0281-0.

Index

D

E

F

G

H

I

J

K

L

M

N

O

T

U

V

W

Y

Z